Reviews for
Addicted: Cold Water Submersion

"The true story of one woman's highly unusual addiction.

Peck Vona dates the beginning of her addiction to cold water to '72, but traces the longer history of her obsessive-compulsive behavior. The physical discomforts and psychological unrest that disrupted her childhood in mid-century upstate New York are keys to understanding her story. A life is a difficult thing to summarize and Peck Vona's is altered by an unheard of addiction and a multitude of shifting obsessions. The author is extremely sensitive to temperature and suffers from feelings of extreme heat that intensify after she eats; as a child and teenager she goes through bouts of self-starvation and bingeing, as an adult she schedules her life around finding places to swim and taking multiple cold showers or ice baths a day. As is often the case with addiction, she distances herself from family, loses jobs and then places to live. The turning point of the book—and of the life upon which it is based—comes when a 31-year-old, malnourished Peck Vona rents a room from a construction laborer named Paul. Paul is there for the lowest points of her addiction and remains with her—as a friend, then lover, then husband—as she slowly frees herself. The book is about a woman becoming physically, as well as figuratively, comfortable in her own skin. The voice that emerges is earnest and can be unexpectedly moving.

A thorough record of sometimes shocking personal fact: a compelling memoir."

Kirkus Discoveries, Kirkus Media LLC, 6411 Burleson Rd., TX 78744

discoveries@kirkusreviews.com

"This is a story of a woman who has dealt with invisible demons, wrecking havoc in her life and decreasing her ability to function. In spite of these intensely isolating obstacles, she has shown resiliency and persistence to persevere toward creating a sense of peace, harmony, and thriving. At the time of this publication, she describes an appreciation and love of life and all it has to offer. This journey can be seen as the eternal spiritual journey of the human soul, into the depth of despair and working its way back to the light. This book should be very insightful for those who are or know someone struggling with obsession, compulsion, and addiction. There IS hope."

Jen Dygert, Eugene Oregon
MSW, LCSW, Mental Health Therapist

"I believe as the author you bring the reader into your home, holding nothing back. We get to know you and your pets and your husband, Paul. The reader also gets a look at how O.C.D. can take over a person's life and personality. How destructive it can be. Paul was very instrumental in helping you with your obsessions. What would have happened if he put his foot down and said enough? We don't know. But what the reader does see is the unconditional love that he has, and his willingness to make Jill feel comfortable in your own skin. He never once says "I can't take this anymore." Instead he asks, "What can I do to help?" I believe, and this is what I believe, that once you accepted Jesus as your Savior you started to see a light at the end of the tunnel. It took some baby steps, and that is okay, but you walked the walk. You show the reader while you are taking those baby steps how, along the way, your life changes little by little. In other words it wasn't like you didn't change until you got through to the light, it changed with every step you took towards it. As a reader I am now towards the end of the book where it shows your sense of humor, peace with yourself, willingness to try new things, not thinking of your needs but the needs of others. It is a truly a wonderful transformation. You have become the Poster Child of what "Normal" is. Allowing the reader to travel the road with you has been an amazing journey and I think anyone who reads it will take a look at their own self and say, "What can I do to improve me?" There are many people out their that have some of the same issues you had, and if after they read the book if only one person sees them self and changes, then the book is a best seller in my eyes."

Elissa Holt, CVA- Porter, Texas

"... is Jill's brutally honest story of her fall into addiction and obsession, and how through courage and a sincere love of life and the undying love and patience of her husband, Paul, drags herself out of the depths of her disease to live a normal life. As a fellow addict I find her book to be another inspiration to continue my own recovery."

Richard Markes, R.N., Albany, New York

"Jill Peck Vona's writing is fearless. She describes an addiction to cold water that most of us could never imagine. And yet, her step by step eloquence about her dive into addiction makes an old story fresh. This is a must read for anyone who needs to understand whatever devil plagues you — for the perspective and the hope for transformation that it gives."

Mally Cox-Chapman - Author, *The Case for Heaven*

"Recovery is an often-misused word in today's vernacular. Bookshelves are full of memoirs of people who have come back from the abyss of addictions. Some are even true stories . . . the story of her struggle with her own body temperature is more than a story of survival and recovery, it is a story of a miracle. The miracle is the power of persistence and love. Some of us are afflicted by the ordinary things in life, too many cocktails becomes the disease of alcoholism. Drugs overpower our moral judgment. Food becomes an obsession . . . the reader learns of the all-consuming ordeal of the author in being comfortable in her own skin. The description of the terror and often agony is moving and compelling.

Intertwined in this story of determination is a love story between Peck-Vona and her husband Paul. The reader shares their unequivocal understanding of each other. The reader senses that these two people have lived their lives together for the joy of each other.

The author is a college-educated artist who's commissioned works have been displayed and sold at auctions in New York City and Albany. She now has given to her readers an artist's view of her unusual struggle against a personal demon. Through the help of medical professionals, her faith and her love she is a success story. This book is a success and will move you and inspire."

James E. Long Esq., Attorney, Albany, New York

ADDICTED:

COLD WATER SUBMERSION

Jill Peck Vona

ADDICTED:

COLD WATER SUBMERSION

Jill Peck Vona

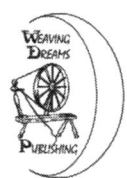

Weaving Dreams Publishing
Watseka, Illinois

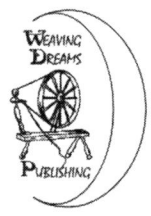

Weaving Dreams Publishing
P. O. Box 194
Watseka, IL 60970

www.weavingdreamspublishing.com

Library of Congress Control Number
2011945792

Cover Art by Kelly Young
© 2009 Kelly Young

Printed in the United States of America
10 9 8 7 6 5 4 3 2

To Paul,
A man with God's unconditional love,
And the patience of Job.

TABLE OF CONTENTS

FOREWORD ONE

I first had contact with Jill in 2006 when she sent me an e-mail about two orphaned newborn kittens she and her husband had found in their garden. I have experience with raising orphaned newborn kittens, and Jill needed some advice on what to do for them. Molly and Duma, as they named the kittens, grew and developed and eventually began to run around and play and to eat on their own. From time to time, Jill e-mailed messages about the kittens and sent me pictures of them.

Then one day, Jill e-mailed to say that she was going to have hip replacement surgery and that she would be offline for a while until she had healed enough to get back to her computer. When Jill was able to e-mail again, she told me she had started writing her book—this book, as it turns out.

After she had finished the manuscript, Jill sent me a copy to read. Her story of addiction to cold water and her obsession for other rituals related to eating (or not eating) is compelling.

It may seem strange that someone could be addicted to something as benign as water. Addictive behaviors, no matter what the person is addicted to, appear remarkably similar. The more I read, the more I wondered how she could have survived what she put herself through.

Jill's story covers her ups and downs, her good days and bad days and, ultimately, her success and triumph in regaining a more normal existence with normal activities. An exceptionally talented woman who is artistic by nature, she has woven a story that takes readers to the depths of her addiction and her obsessions and brings them back up into the light and the love that she eventually discovered.

Jill unselfishly shares her story of hope and faith in God and love for the "angel here on earth" who rescued her from herself and in time became her husband. Through her book, she reaches out to those who are suffering and to those who love someone who is suffering. Her courage in dealing with her problems—and in reaching out to others—is an inspiration for us all.

Author and Journalist   LeAnn R. Ralph
Colfax, Wisconsin

FOREWORD TWO

When Jill Peck Vona asked me if I would like to read the draft of her book, *Addicted to Cold Water*, I responded that, of course, I would.

Little did I know of the impact that this personal and courageous account of her life and struggles would have on me. Although we had been close childhood friends, we went our separate ways after high school and lost touch until some forty years later, coinciding with a high school reunion and my need to visit a doctor very close in proximity to Jill's residence. Our friendship was rekindled, and I have tried to visit her as often as possible, even if only for a quick hug and thirty minutes of catching up.

In our early teens, we spent a great deal of time in each other's homes, which seemed the natural progression given that our parents were best friends, and Jill and I were classmates. I always thought the Pecks enjoyed the most ideal family situation and never would have guessed, or predicted, the underlying and insidious struggles invading the very core of Jill's existence.

Throughout the years, from time to time, I heard mention of Jill's life, either from my parents or others who knew of her, alluding to problems she was having and a lifestyle that was both troubling and hard to believe, given the illusion of such normalcy in earlier years. Hints at eating disorders and not dressing appropriately for the harsh winter weather were shared, but never in detail and devoid of an explanation as to the cause of this behavior.

Not until we renewed our communication did the picture start to unfold for me, and it filled me with both deep sadness and horror that such a "normal," kind, caring, and loving person would have to endure such a torturous existence.

Once I started reading *Addicted to Cold Water*, I found myself mesmerized and picked it up whenever I had a few free moments. Of course, part of that stemmed from the bond of an old friendship and the natural curiosity of what had transpired, but mostly it was the vulnerable honesty with which Jill tells her story, which is both deeply painful and triumphant. Her struggles put into perspective how trivial most of our "problems" are and how we so easily take for granted our day-to-day routines, simple things that we barely think about, but for her have been major obstacles and have consumed her every waking thought.

I certainly have a newfound and profound respect for the author of this, a chronicle of an often-crippling and tortured life, and feel certain it will not only inspire but also help to heal those with similar struggles. I am proud to call Jill Peck Vona my friend; I salute her husband, Paul, for saving her life; I commend her for this tough labor of love; and congratulate her on the huge strides she has made to enjoy a life in which she takes great pride in kicking the monsters of her past out her front door and welcoming hope and joy in their place.

Legal Assistant   Allyson Sorge
New York, 2012

PREFACE

I want to share my story so that anyone can see there is always   hope of a better tomorrow even when you have an addiction. My addiction was to cold water, and it took over my life. The current that pulled me under was strong and demanding. At times, getting out of the perilous hole I was in put me on a very slippery slope. I slid backward occasionally, but I never gave up and always had a very strong will to live no matter what it took.

This book starts out on a high note when I thought I had the world by the tail, as an employee at McCall's Pattern in New York City. It follows the downward spiral fall that left me very ill with a temperature of eighty-eight degrees and weighing in at a little over one hundred pounds, five feet nine inches. The story unfolds into a journey back to health and a wonderful love story with a fantastic, caring man.

I have tried numerous times to write this book and set it aside. I had to have a hip replacement in 2006. When I came home from the hospital, it was easier to be on the lower level of our house, not where the computer was located, of course. So, instead of sitting at a computer doing my usual, I began to journal in the evening. I was relaxed with nothing else on my mind. It was quiet, and I was alone. The words just flowed out easily. I have still revised it several times since then. This final version begins with my summer in New York City and moves back to my childhood and young adulthood, and the period of time when my obsessions, compulsions, and addiction began.

This is what I have wanted to tell: how I went from being, for the most part, normal to someone so hot I couldn't take being indoors for any length of time, especially to eat. I turned to swimming in cold water and taking ice baths for what I thought was my chance for survival. I became so ill and thin that I was diagnosed with anorexia and hypothermia.

With the punishment my body endured, it's a wonder I am still alive. I damaged myself physically and mentally, and I ended up with a body temperature that will not stay constant. In the process of attempting recovery, I attached myself to many new obsessions or mini-addictions, which allowed me to slowly move forward. I rationalized my situation and concluded that each one was a little less destructive, bringing me closer to a fuller life.

The journey to heal was long: thirty years plus. In the beginning, if someone would have told me I would become a happy, independent woman capable of standing on my own two feet, run a household indoors and out, and that I would be married, I would never have believed them. I knew in my heart I wasn't going to die. Anything beyond that was in God's hands. Looking back, I realized that even when I didn't know he was with me, I truly believe he was carrying me to my destination.

It has taken years and years to make a halfway-normal comeback to a lifestyle that most people would accept. I still struggle on some days. I am never totally sure if some parts of my addictive behavior are still with me. I have kicked the addiction to frigid cold. A lower-than-average body temperature has lingered along with minor fears, migraines, and a very limited social life.

Addictions and obsessive-compulsive behaviors consume anyone who suffers from them. I hope reading my story makes you feel not as alone as you find your path to recovery. Learning about your body, trying to stay positive, looking to God in those moments of very deep despair, and giving yourself time to heal is my best advice. If you can find someone to love you unconditionally, and who has faith in you, as I did, your odds of improvement increase.

May God bless you all as you take each daily step.

Latham, New York   JPV
March, 2012

ACKNOWLEDGMENTS

I am forever grateful to my editor/publisher Sue Durkin, for her encouragement, patience, and talent.

Eternally thankful to my late mother and father, Jean and Buel Peck, who dedicated themselves to giving me a happy childhood full of love and respect. Because of their guidance, I am not one to give up easily.

Thanks to my art teachers, Mrs. Barbara Lynch and Professor David Broudo. They gave me the gift of loving the arts and the inspiration to be forever creative. It was their foundation that help build a network of many versatile artistic interests, which I have drawn upon throughout my healing years.

Thanks to the late Sonna Calendrino, who welcomed me with open arms at one of the lowest points in my life.

Deep gratitude to Sheila Eustace for giving me shelter from the storm, when I had nowhere else to go. I believe God placed her in my path for a reason. She was the bridge that led me to a brighter tomorrow, and to my future husband.

Thanks to my stepson Arthur Vona, who respected my illness and my addiction. He brought me to a place where I am able to accept people working around me at mealtimes.

Special thanks to my sister-friend, Susie Sunshine, who helped me to let go of the things I can't control.

I am forever grateful to LeAnn Ralph for all the hours spent correcting my first manuscript. And who inspired me to continue writing with gusto. I couldn't have written this book without her.

And to my friend, Valerie Vautrin, who, after my second surgery, was my aide and companion. With her by my side, I was able to dismiss a long-standing habit, which had interfered with a normal life style for too many years.

A thank you to Glenn and Scottie, the contractors who renovated the outside of our home during the winter months of 2007. In order to complete each stage of the project the contractors needed my approval. I had sheltered myself from the cold, mostly out of fear. I needed to move on, and because of them, I endured the cold outdoors much longer than I thought possible. They gave me a wonderful gift: more freedom.

March, 2012   Jill Peck Vona
New York

The Story

Of

My Addiction

Chapter 1
The Kiddy Pool

If someone asked me a few years ago, "Do you believe in Heaven and Hell?" I would have certainly answered, "Absolutely. I am living in Hell right now."

There is heat, and then there is *hot*. If Hell is like this, then I pray I don't ever go there. Every day, the pressure that pushed down upon my body was oppressive. There seemed to be little I could do to get relief. Each morning, there was the same thing to look forward to: try to survive the heat that burned deep into every part of my body.

I finally settled in a nice neighborhood. Latham, New York wasn't overly populated, and it appeared to be a peaceful town. I rarely spoke to anyone because I was too wrapped up in my dilemma. The neighbors went about their business; I kept to myself, for the most part. Paul was my landlord at the time. He had no clue as to what I was enduring. I tried to act human while suffering with something I couldn't control.

Only when I was asleep, did the torture subside. As soon as one eye opened, I felt the heat engulf the top of my head, work its way to my neck, continue down my torso, and finish at my feet, as if following a map. This daily pattern was a thorn in my side — a depressing existence. With the heat keeping me a prisoner most of the day, I had no appetite. Whatever I thought I might be able to consume, my body told me otherwise as soon as it entered the blood stream. I dreaded eating; it was too difficult.

On one particular morning in July, I decided it was time to make a change. There had to be a temporary solution. I couldn't take it anymore. My mind raced in all directions, looking for an answer. I had to get rid of the awful heat that raged throughout my body. I had no peace. Heat and fear was all I felt each time I looked at food. No matter what I consumed, the heat escalated. I wanted to live more than anything, yet I dreaded each day. I was trapped inside my own hot body.

In desperation, I persuaded Paul to go out and buy me a kiddy pool and several bags of ice. I put the plastic pool in my bedroom! Yes, in my bedroom. And he let me do it.

I was embarrassed to let anyone see my ritual. Bathing in ice behind closed doors made it seem more acceptable. I didn't want any interference during the process. Once I started with the cooling down procedure, any interruption might inhibit the cold I was receiving from the treatment. And a tightly closed door would keep all the cold in one spot.

I'm fairly certain most landlords don't allow a pool in a bedroom. Paul saw how miserable I was, and he just wanted to help a young girl who, apparently, was in trouble. He didn't have to understand it at the time.

I didn't rationalize what ice would do to my body. My only thought was to, finally, be cool enough to eat. The anticipation and excitement of having all that cold around me was awesome. It brought me back to the days of swimming in very cold water. Now I knew I would be able to eat enough to stay healthy and happy.

Before each meal, I filled the kiddy pool with water and at least, one bag of ice. The coldness instantly shot up to my knees as I stepped into the frigid water. I smiled with relief as this heavenly feeling soothed my skin. Standing in frosty, cold water and ice cubes, I took a washcloth and covered myself with the ice water from head to toe. Not just once, but over and over again. It was as if I were layering my entire body in degrees of cold. The more layers there were, the longer the cold would last, spreading throughout my body and numbing every inch of my soul until I felt nothing on the exterior. My numb fingers made it difficult to hold the washcloth, but I had to have more of the cold. Wanting more and more, I was like a junkie looking for a fix. The best part was feeling the icy, cold water run over my head. I closed my eyes and enjoyed the cold as it transformed a gray day into one with millions of rainbows. As the water rushed over my skull and down my eyelids, I felt the pressure release in my head. All the heat I felt escaped out into the air like the top being taken off a kettle of boiling water. I opened my eyes with a new vision and clarity that made my life so much happier. The cold gave me a euphoric high, sending my brain into another world. My appetite was enormous, and all my senses awakened. I felt beautiful and alive.

The very thing destroying me was what I craved most: icy water. And, because it wasn't cold enough, I asked Paul to install an air conditioner. I wanted to contain as much cold within my body as possible.

Returning to my ice-cold paradise was what I looked forward to each day. It was there, where I found freedom once again. I was away from the world that didn't understand. I found sanity within these cold walls. I was released from the pain; the heat that swelled up inside my body was gone.

The cold bedroom didn't accept the water treatment as well as I did. I was too numb to notice. The water on the floor removed the heavy, poly finish right down to the bare wood. A veneer vanity, in perfect condition, rippled and became unglued in various places. The edges loosened and buckled up on the rest of the furniture, and the mirror was covered with droplets of water that eventually warped the wood frame. The calendar on the wall curled up so that the month wasn't visible, the walls glistened when any light hit the moisture that formed on the surface, and green mold grew in the corners of the room. All of this resulted from too much cold water.

Paul knew I was using ice; he just didn't know the extent of it. I closed the door so no one could see the amount of ice I had in the pool or how long I bathed in it. I was heading downhill. At the time, I didn't even think what was happening. I had to eat in order to stay alive. If ice, cold water and an air conditioner gave me what I needed, then, as far as I was concerned, this was my only option; and there was no discussing it. I was living in an ice world.

I couldn't prepare my meals and stay cold at the same time. The home aide still came to the house. When it was time to eat, I entered my bedroom and, literally, tried to freeze myself. As soon as I became too hot, there was no eating, so the aide prepared my meal.

When I was close to *dead* cold, I hollered from the doorway, "Okay, I'm ready to eat."

The aide brought my meal up and handed it to me in the doorway. I ate as fast as I could before I became hot again. I repeated this procedure three times a day.

There was a time in my life when my lifestyle brought about a low, body temperature. It was happening again. I was too overtaken with heat to think rational. I just reacted to being too warm, and the ice-cold water felt good on my hot skin. Summer helped keep me out of the hospital. After leaving my freezing bedroom, the rest of the house felt extremely warm. The interlude of occasional heat probably helped my body temperature from staying too low for too long.

Paul knew something was up, but he let me continue throughout the summer. Returning each day from work, he found me closed in my room, bathing in ice-cold water. He saw a woman in severe trouble, and he felt helpless. He didn't want to lose me.

I wouldn't listen to reason. My way of existing and stubbornness took me back into the darkness. The addiction took over once again.   Paul was very sad as he witnessed this obsessive behavior. Finally, after watching this sequence of events for several months, he couldn't stand by and do nothing. He went to the nearby community, health center where I previously saw a doctor. My doctor wasn't working that day. The one on call was a psychiatrist.

The psychiatrist said, "Take the ice away. Eventually, Jill will eat."

Paul came home and did just that.

I remember the day as if it were yesterday. I just finished bathing and was in the middle of my lunch. Paul opened my door and took the kiddy pool out of the room — ice water and all. Balancing the kiddy pool as best he could,

Paul walked down the stairs, and then threw it out the front door.

I was in a state of shock. I thought someone had stopped me from breathing. I couldn't believe what just happened. I never expected him to enter my room without asking. It was so bold and aggressive. I was stunned beyond words. When I comprehended the reality, I begged him to bring the pool back, but he refused. My heart sank. I was angry, scared, and felt sick to my stomach. My security was just demolished. I couldn't even look at Paul. I felt betrayed and hurt.

My first thought was, "I will not eat if I don't have ice."

Two doors down from my bedroom was a smaller room. I went there, lay down, and cried myself to sleep.

Chapter 2
Early Years

If you asked me when my addiction to cold water definitely started, I would say 1972, although there were warning signs much earlier. The obsessive-compulsive behavior that controlled me was responding to an overwhelming feeling of body heat. The need to cool down was already placing limitations on my actions and restricting my life. I knew it, but never before shared my difficulties with anyone. Even I had no clue how devastating the situation would, eventually, become.

Summers in New York can get pretty warm, and most families head to the water to cool off. In 1950, when I was three years old, Dad and my uncle built the family cabin on Copake Lake in Columbia County, New York. Right up until my late twenties, I was fortunate to have this haven during the hot, summer months.

In the early part of May, Mom aired out and cleaned the cabin, in preparation of the summer ahead. As soon as school ended, we packed our summer clothes and moved to the lake. Once we were situated, I was content, unless a great movie was playing at the cinema in town. In my eyes, the lake was a paradise; it was my most favorite spot in the world.

I don't remember being a baby. However, my assumption was, and is, the most important things at that time in my life were food, sleep, and love. By the time I was five, going to the lake was close in importance.

Some of my earliest memories are of kindergarten. They come back to me in bits and pieces like a jigsaw puzzle scattered about on a table. The winter season was the most difficult. I wasn't in love with wearing layers of heavy clothing that made me too hot. I had a poor attention span, and the heat of the classroom intensified that drowsy feeling.

Drawing pictures was probably my favorite time in school. However, the big fat pencil, which always had a dull point, upset me. I thought, how could anyone do good work with an unsharpened pencil? And why didn't the teacher, at the beginning of each class, see to it that all the pencil points were neatly filed? I also enjoyed helping out in the kitchen for juice and cracker break and talking with the lady in charge.

Spring was the best time when all the windows were open, and we went out to the playground.

I lived within walking distance of the *little school* and, because I enjoyed the exercise and being with my mother, I came home every day for lunch.

Of course, the highlight of the year was still our summer vacation at the lake.

Daddy taught me how to swim when I was four. Now there I was very comfortable, and I did excel. As I gained confidence, my strokes were near perfection, which I strived for at a young age. Even now, it is important to point out the issue of perfection. My dad also taught me how to snow ski at the age of six and to water ski when I was twelve. I struggled to become flawless, never reaching my goal.

In 1959, Mom and Dad bought a sailfish, a new experience for us all. (sailfish- a flat sailboat introduced in the late 1950's. It provided an easy way to learn how to sail. The sailor sat on the flat deck and placed his or her feet in a footwell. Then he or she held the rope to the sail with one hand, and the other hand held the rutter.) The first time I went with my father, it was a hot, sunny day, with a crystal-clear blue sky and a moderate breeze. As the boat tilted to one side, Dad told me to lean out over the water. Our bodies kept the sail from flipping her over. It was amazing. I wanted more windy days, but only hot ones. Even though heat bothered me most of the time, as long as I could jump into the lake, at any given time, I was fine.

There were days when I gazed out over the lake, and the waves had a white tip, which usually meant the wind was coming out of the north. A north wind is much cooler, especially on the water. Those days weren't for me; I always ended up with a very bad headache. However, those waves were the most challenging, and it killed me to sit them out. I checked the temperature gauge — over and over — as if, by some great feat, that would make it climb upward. I tried to control that, too.

When I was very young, many of my dresses were hand sewn with beautiful and intricate smocking on the front bodices, which involved patience and devotion. Then my mother made an exact duplicate of my dress for my doll. She either made our Halloween outfits, or we went to the attic, and she put together an outfit as if by magic.

Mom taught me how to sew, knit, cook, and perform other household chores. I followed her directions, but my creations weren't perfect. I needed her close by, in case I screwed up. I never felt I measured up to her talents and expertise, except in the kitchen. I enjoyed making many kinds of homemade cookies and being creative with salad dressings.

From a very young age, what I wanted out of my life was to be just like my mother, plus accomplish as much in life as my father.

I grew up in a very loving family. I was too protected from the real world, but I always felt I could depend upon home as a safe haven. No matter what issues occurred away from the family, I knew everything was okay when we were together.

I wanted so much to please my parents in every aspect of my life, both at home and in school. I thought they were perfect, and I looked up to them as role models. It appeared to me that they lived every part of their day faultlessly. They were caring and understanding, and spent so much time with my sister and me. They gave of themselves each day in order to make us happy.

In all of my attempts to emulate them, I never really considered that it took them years to develop the skill and poise they exhibited by the time I joined their lives. The expectations I put on myself, to be just like them from an early age, put me in a perfect position to fail at many of my attempts. That, in turn, reinforced my desire to succeed and, quite possibly, instigated my obsessive-compulsive behavior.

I wasn't at all prepared for the change that came. Some of the problems that became serious issues later in my life began to surface in small ways at a very young age.

Until I was seven years of age, my mother braided my hair every morning. I always sat in the same chair near the kitchen sink so she could access the water, which was needed to keep the strands of hair together. She meticulously created two perfect braids and placed them securely on top of my head. The braids were flawless with every hair in place. I looked forward to this perfect scene and routine every day before school.

One morning, she informed me that I was old enough to learn how to braid my own hair. I was devastated. I knew I couldn't braid it like she did. I didn't want to go to school, and I continued to dwell on this horrible moment in my life. Why did she stop braiding my hair? My best friend's mother still braided her hair. I was mad. I felt as if my school days would never be the same. I did continue to attend, but I wasn't happy about my hair. Whatever I did with it, I wasn't pleased with the outcome. My hair was certainly an intermittent issue throughout my life.

In the early '50s, we began taking Sunday rides as a family. We often went to visit relatives. One, in particular, was a wonderful cook and baker. Her kitchen smelled of cinnamon and everything homemade. It was warm, cozy, and perfectly country. There was always a pie or cake and lots of cookies on hand.

I always felt uneasy when asked to sample a delightful dessert. As far back as I can remember, I was concerned about eating the high-calorie foods, followed by a long time of sitting in a warm house. I was afraid of overheating without a way to cool off. And then there was always the weight gain that forever pressed upon my brain, so all I could do was mitigate any damages and not eat.

I remember, at a young age, when hors d'oeuvres were served. They always looked so enticing. Mommy made chicken liver pate, which was one of my favorites. After eating it, I wished I hadn't. Once I started, it was very difficult to stop. Fresh, cold shrimp with cocktail sauce was another one. Next, came the big dinner, and after digesting all of that food, I felt miserably warm and a bit larger in size. I hated myself for overindulging. The heat should have disappeared or not bothered me, but it seemed to last forever. So much so, I dwelled on how I felt for the rest of the day.

Each time I gave in to this *extra eating*, I promised myself: never again. Yet, when there was another occasion, holiday, or evening out for dinner, with plenty of my favorite foods, I fell back into the party element and gave in.

Around 1959, I became a member of the 4-H. My first summer as a member, I begged my parents to let me go camp. They agreed. I had visions of lush, green grass and beautiful surroundings–of buildings with open windows where a warm, summer breeze blew gently across the room, keeping it a comfortable temperature. I saw myself sitting in a dining hall with a huge fan blowing to keep the room comfortable. And children sat at the tables, laughing and enjoying the usual summertime, favorite meals.

As I sat in the family car, and Dad drove closer to the camp, my visions faded. The scenery was far from pleasant. I had a lump in my throat, and my chest tightened with fear. That feeling intensified to dread when I saw the camp. It was dreary and dull with dead shrubs and a few old buildings. The land was dry and full of weeds. It didn't look like a camp. It didn't look like fun.

At that moment, I definitely knew I didn't want to be there. It was devil-dreadful hot. To top it off, there was no pond or lake. I felt instantly sick, and all I wanted to do was head straight home.

Mom and Dad said I made a commitment, and I had to stick with it. I was mortified and mad at them; however, they wouldn't give in to my plea.

The meals made me nauseous. The smells and the heat in the dining hall took my appetite away. At home, we ate fresh fruits and vegetables, wheat bread and salad; and rather simple dishes of chicken, fish, or meat. The food at camp was mixed-up concoctions and unfamiliar tastes that didn't digest well. I ate very little and counted the days until departure time.

All we did throughout the day was work on silly crafts in the heat. All I wanted to do was cool off in cold water. I was never so happy to leave a place.

I did learn a lesson: when I commit to something, it is important to finish it through.

Soon after that, Mom started a Girl Scout troop. I was hesitant about going to their summer camp. It had a lake, and that helped in my decision. At first, I missed Copake Lake, but once I was in the swing of things, I loved it. Camp Little Notch was located north of Albany, New York. I returned there for, at least, five more summers. The only things I didn't like were the warm, dining hall and the food. The food was foreign to my usual diet. My body reacted the same as it did at 4-H camp. Once again, the big, bad monster followed me: the predicament of how and what to eat in order to stay cool.

I often found myself snacking on candy bars. Sometimes the urge was so bad, I couldn't stop eating them, but I didn't want anyone to see me; so I took them to bed at night and ate them secretly in the dark. The cool, night air made it easier for me to consume the high-calorie food. But the next day, I felt terribly hot from all the sugar.

Other than that, Girl Scout camp left me with wonderful memories. Each time we arrived back in Albany, we all cried. We were glad to see our parents and sad to leave our friends. Mom and Dad never knew if I was happy to see them.

The trip back to Copake took over an hour, and I don't think I came up for air once. I had plenty to talk about after two weeks of camp. I never shared my food or candy issues with my parents, though. When I was back home with my family, only the happy memories were important.

Scouting was a sacred part of my life, and Mom was always my leader. In 1962, I was chosen   —   along with seven other girls from different neighboring troops   —   to attend the Girl Scout Roundup in Button Bay, Vermont, as a consolidated troop from our region. Just because we were chosen, it didn't mean the decision couldn't be reversed. We had to prove we were worthy.

There was a preliminary event   —   kind of a practice session for the real thing — held at the Girl Scout camps in East Greenbush, New York. Our troop had to put up tents in record time and present our demonstration. Each troop going to the roundup had to have a demonstration, which told something about the area they came from.

My troop wasn't organized: we didn't really know one another, we couldn't get the tents up properly, and even our knots were tied wrong. Heaven forbid, if a bad storm came along, everything would be lost. We didn't have a demonstration in mind, and nothing went right. The scout leader in charge of the event said we wouldn't be going to the roundup if we didn't get our act together, and quickly. My mother happened to be at the same campground with her troop. I was close to tears when I walked into her campsite.

She calmed me down and said, "Take a deep breath. We'll figure something out." She didn't have the answer at the moment.

I returned the following day. While I waited for Mom to finish up with her own troop, a member, and good friend of mine, told me something very shocking. I learned that my strong-willed, multitasking mother, who I believed could take on the world and help anyone with his or her problems, picked up smoking after quitting for eleven years. I couldn't believe me ears. I kept asking, "Are you sure? But why?" Later on, I learned it was from the stressful weekend. I felt horrible that I did this to her. At the time, the minutes were ticking away toward the deadline of who was going to the roundup, and our desperation took priority.

Mom asked the head leader if she would give our troop one weekend to improve and show we were ready, and her request was approved. Mom told us we were going to meet at our cabin on Copake Lake the next weekend and figure this mess out. We did just that. She drilled us — over and over — until we were putting up tents in record time.

We still needed something for our demonstration, though. Mom suggested we look into the Hudson Valley and its history. It didn't take us long to realize there was a lot of potential with the Indians from that region. We made two deerskin outfits and purchased moccasins, necklaces, and two black wigs to give our models an authentic look. Our research led us to information about wampum, and we decided to have our *Indians* weave a wampum belt for our demonstration.

Because of my mother, our troop passed with flying colors, and we were on our way to the roundup.

As much as I loved being a Girl Scout, I disliked the material of the green uniform. It was stiff and warm, and very uncomfortable. When I became a Mariner Girl Scout, my mother surprised me with a handsome, blue uniform. I would have gladly worn it as a daily outfit. The material was soft and didn't overheat my skin. I also felt special wearing it. The almost *military look* made a statement of importance.

If you looked behind the *little school* — that is what we called the grade school, kindergarten though third grade — you would never find me stealing a kiss from a boy. I couldn't even talk to the opposite sex without my face turning a crimson color. I was never sure of what to say or what to do in order to make an impression. This feeling followed me into adulthood.

I took ballroom dancing when I was thirteen. I wanted to dance as well as my parents. I was thrilled whenever my father asked me to dance, but I was extremely nervous. I was afraid of making a mistake. I was never relaxed when I learned a new step or anything new. How could I be, when I placed impossible demands for immediate perfection upon myself? I thought I fell short of what was expected of me, regardless of any compliments.

At high school mixers, I envied my classmates as I watched them dance. They made it look so easy. I fumbled my way through each dance, frustrated that I didn't show more expertise. I went alone to all the mixers. At the beginning of each new song, my hopes were high, but I *sat out* most dances.

Dating wasn't something I longed for. I didn't go steady in high school or wear a guy's ring around my neck. I liked high school — don't get me wrong — I just wasn't popular. I had friends, but I still spent most of my leisure time with my parents.

I took piano lessons from 1956-1963, for longer than I want to remember. I thought it would be wonderful to just sit down and play. Whenever I heard a pianist, I was mesmerized. I was sure, with practice, I would eventually play quite well. However, I dreaded the long lessons and the boring scales. The heat in the house swelled my fingers. I nervously reached for each key, hoping it was the right one. As I stumbled through the hour, hoping it would end soon, my jovial, warm-hearted teacher patiently waited for me to finish. Always emphasizing to practice more, but never making me feel any less of a human being. Her cocker spaniel was adorable. He probably stayed close by because he was deaf.

Throughout my childhood and teen years, my parents encouraged my interests and helped me develop them and any talent I exhibited. Yet, in spite of all the encouragement and acknowledgment for my accomplishments, I felt inferior. I put myself down for not being the best at whatever I tried to do. I was adequate, but that wasn't good enough for me. I never felt I lived up to my potential.

I had some achievements during my teen years. From 1963 to 1965, during Christmas breaks, I was a ski bum in Vermont (a person who waits tables, normally at a ski lodge, plus obtains a free, ski pass). My high school coach asked me to attend a lifeguard school in Pennsylvania. This qualified me for a lifeguard position and a swimming instructor. I was crowned senior, prom queen in 1965. Then I made dean's list while attending Endicott Jr. College.

I'm sure you are wondering how I mastered the different activities that I've mentioned thus far. There were many wonderful days throughout this period, but the years didn't pass without discomfort due to the extra heat I felt within my body. I asked myself why. That's as far as my question went. I assumed I had to live with it.

At social gatherings, I never sampled anything and allowed myself to feel uncomfortable because I was sure people were talking about me and wondering why I never tasted any food. Once the festivities were over, I acted like it didn't matter, until the next holiday or party came along. Unfortunately, I felt safe in my comfort zone and missed out on some parts of a typical, teenage life.

When friends and relatives invited our family to dinner, I dreaded going. First of all, I couldn't decide what to wear. I wanted to wear a stylish outfit, but not one that overheated me. I decided on an outfit, and once I was in the car, I wished I had worn something else. Then I worried about what kind of food would be served. The clothing I wore, plus the food I ate — how would I feel afterward? I watched everyone else carry on and enjoy the evening. I squirmed in my skin and couldn't wait to go home. I pretended to enjoy myself. I guess I was a good actress.

My mother's menu was quite different from the food served at social gatherings and at school. I was used to Mom's cooking, and I tolerated it quite well. Occasionally, she made an angel food cake. It was Dad's favorite — and mine, too. The cake was complete when the nice, butter frosting was added. Every time I walked past the cake, my craving grew stronger. I resisted for as long as I could. Usually, I indulged in the evening after everyone was in bed. That way, if I suffered, I was alone. A nice, cold glass of milk made the combination wonderful and briefly compensated for any heat in my body, obtained from the ingredients. But as soon as the sugar hit the blood stream, the heat intensified. Then I was mad at myself for eating it. I was jealous that other people could eat anything and not be affected. As a teen, I felt I was the only one with a crisis, and one I couldn't fix.

Many foods *stoked up the fire* in my body: frosted cakes or pies, hot chocolate, ice cream, whipped cream, candy, marshmallow topping, hot fudge, most store-bought cookies — especially Oreos, Italian sausage, pizza, lasagna, French fries, meatballs, and gravy, to name a few.

As a child, when playing at my best friend's house, Oreos were the favorite cookie. After eating only one, my whole body felt like I stepped into a sauna, especially my face. It flushed a vivid pink. I was miserable and uncomfortable as I continued to play with my friends. In time, the heat lessened, but I was always glad to return home.

I had some achievements during my teen years. From 1963 to 1965, during Christmas breaks, I was a ski bum in Vermont (a person who waits tables, normally at a ski lodge, plus obtains a free, ski pass). My high school coach asked me to attend a lifeguard school in Pennsylvania. This qualified me for a lifeguard position and a swimming instructor. I was crowned senior, prom queen in 1965. Then I made dean's list while attending Endicott Jr. College.

As I mentioned earlier, in my childhood days, certain foods contributed to the heat I felt. This didn't change when I became a teenager. I loved pizza, but the reaction was the same. Every Labor Day, my friends and I dressed up in silly outfits and went to a local pizzeria via our motorboat. This tradition was our way of ending the summer.

I wanted to be a part of the group and to be liked by my friends, so I went along. I knew what the reaction would be — similar to someone being allergic, I guess. I didn't want to be the oddball or announce why I'd rather not eat pizza. No one would understand; more than likely, my friends would laugh. It was also one of my fears at pajama parties; what food would be served? The heat I felt separated me from my friends. I felt different.

When I was young, the problem wasn't as severe as later on. I still carried on, living my day in a normal way; my vital signs were good, and no one was the wiser. Whatever I was feeling, I never discussed it with my mother. When it came to food and heat, I just didn't fit in.

In high school, I was voted best dressed. I spent a lot of time and energy deciding what to wear each day. Every school night, I paced back and forth in my walk-in closet. I couldn't go to sleep until I decided on the perfect outfit for the following day. And every morning, I changed my mind again. The skirt didn't go with the top. The colors were wrong. The material made me hot. The skirt was too short or too long. I didn't look pretty. I took so long trying to decide what to wear as I changed one outfit for another and fussed with my hair that I missed the bus many times. During the school day, if the garment wasn't satisfactory it *bugged me* all day until I got home and removed it. Unfortunately, if someone had told me I was preoccupied with a style obsession, I wouldn't have listened. I had created a monster, which, in turn, added more nervous tension than was necessary. It was actually stressful to be stylish, especially with phobias.

Appearance didn't stop with my clothes; my hair and ears were an issue as well. From the time I was very young, I thought my ears stuck out like Dumbo's. With every hairstyle I wore, I tried to cover my ears. As I compared my ears to my girlfriends, I wanted mine to be like theirs, nice and tight to my head. I purchased special glue. I was sure this was my answer to looking pretty. The glue worked. Shortly after the application, my ears itched, and because it was a foreign matter and didn't belong there, I peeled the glue off a little at a time. I was never really satisfied with my appearance until I was a junior in high school. And because of this, I spent my energies in the wrong areas.

When I was a sophomore, a friend invited me to her birthday party. It was a hot, summer day. I probably changed my clothes more times than I want to remember. I was afraid the other girls would giggle or talk about how I looked. I thought the blouse made me look fat. I was sure I'd overheat even before I arrived at the party. I was ready to come home before I left the house.

I viewed my body daily and was my own worst critic on appearance, especially body size. At times, no matter what I put on, I was hot. Not a wonder, with all the exercise I got changing my clothes. Even without the exertion, certain materials made me squirm. I reacted almost instantly. My mood changed. I was totally preoccupied and obsessed with finding the perfect garment where I felt cool. The more I worked at it, the more frustrated I got. I had a mental block against being too warm, yet I emotionally created a terrible amount of heat inside my head just from the stress of it all. As far as I was concerned, these days only had one way of ending — a disaster.

Sex was never discussed when I was growing up. I didn't know about erections, orgasms, protection, and what was expected during intercourse. As a teenager, I never understood any sex jokes. I laughed at them just to fit in with everyone else.

When I was a teenager, I was invited to my best friend's slumber party. The other girls knew all about sex. I was embarrassed that I knew nothing. In the dark, by flashlight, they read the good parts of *Lady Chatterley's Lover*. After the PJ party, I told a few other friends what we read, just to make an impression. That was about the extent of my *sex education*, which left me feeling rather insecure. What we do as teenagers to fit in.

From kindergarten to twelfth grade, plus two years in college, art was my favorite class. It allowed the creative part of my brain to bloom. At the end of each year, we had a colorful, art show. It displayed the talent of many, young students. After Dad viewed mine, I patiently waited for his reaction and hoped it would be positive, and it always was.

Dad probably gave birth to the artistic muse within me, so his critique became extremely import. I was focused when I was at the drawing board, and my grade was consistently excellent. I only had to walk into the art room, and my self-esteem improved. I believe my artistic skills grew with the nurturing of my father and a wonderful art teacher.

Mom and Dad shared their talents, whether it was in the arts and crafts or in sports. I had the interest and the desire to learn. My parents were strong advocates of creativity, and I believe that was more beneficial to me — when I was healthy or ill — than being a bookworm.

I didn't decide on art as my future career, even though I had evidence of talent. I pulled an A every semester of my last two years of high school. Even with all the recognition, I still felt mediocre next to my classmates and convinced myself that I wasn't good enough to continue in any field of art. I concluded a more lucrative career should definitely be considered.

I turned my dream toward becoming a nurse. Unfortunately, I failed chemistry in 1962 and felt my only option was to terminate those hopes. Whatever occupation the guidance counselor suggested, and in spite of all the encouragement and acknowledgment for my accomplishments, I gave him many reasons why I shouldn't pursue any of the careers he mentioned. I put myself down for not being the best at whatever I tried to do.

The days moved along, and I didn't have a career or a college in mind. Whenever I was scheduled to see the guidance counselor, I acquired a horrible, tension headache. My future looked rather bleak and empty for a while.

I ask myself now if I was so set on *perfection* that I sabotaged myself in my attempts or if there was something medical going on I didn't know about.

I attended college from 1965 to 1967. I'm not sure why I majored in retailing, except that I felt I could pass; it was a safe choice. A passing grade was important. However, when I made the dean's list, I believe my parents were as surprised and happy as I was.

I rarely ate in the college, dining hall. As soon as my feet hit the carpet, I knew the temperature was wrong. I felt as if the room was closing in and warm air was swirling all around my head, suffocating me. The hair on my head felt singed, right down to the roots. The clothes on my back felt heavy and prickly. It was difficult to breathe and get enough air. My hands and feet swelled, and my shoes felt too small. I almost had a panic attack when I realized this would be my dining area for the next two years.

I was relieved to find a campus snack shop in the same building. It was on the lower floor and near the entrance. This was more comfortable because there seemed to be some movement of air, and the layout created a feeling of openness.

Nights, when I washed my hair, my roommate brought food back to the dorm room for me. I purchased a lot of tuna fish salad and coffee ice cream. Eating in my room worked out quite well. I was able to stay in one environment without too many temperature changes. When I was ready to eat, someone brought it to me. The items I ordered were always cold. I didn't overeat — just enough to satisfy the taste buds and take away the hunger pains. Between the coffee shop and my bedroom, I managed, so I didn't dwell on my problem or really acknowledge it was a serious issue. I just accepted it. Mom and Dad wondered why I needed so much extra spending money. A good deal of it went to the snack shop.

Throughout the warmer months, the college held cookouts on the beach. These events were not my favorite thing. I dreaded going because I never ate, and being among my classmates with nothing on my plate was embarrassing. I preferred to eat indoors and at the snack shop. The temperatures were more stable, and my skin felt better. If I ate anything outdoors and walked back into a building, I didn't adjust to the temperature change and, therefore, became extremely hot. It was as though my skin was programmed to rebel against the outdoor elements while I ate. When this occurred, it was as if the extra heat I felt was lodged inside my head, and it couldn't get out.

Every time a birthday rolled around, the whole dorm celebrated in what we called the *butt* room. The girls surprised me with a wonderful birthday cake. I didn't eat any, but I had a good time. I politely told my classmates I wasn't hungry, and I'd save a piece of cake for later. Of course, that never happened. The *butt* room was always warm and sometimes stuffy. If I added food, especially sugar, to that, I was sure I'd overheat. I justified the situation by saying that people could have a good time at a party without indulging in food. The gathering wasn't all about food. It was a time to be with friends and to celebrate one's birth or the occasion.

Weight and warmth were a constant battle. For those reasons, I made up my mind to only eat at mealtime. That was difficult enough to keep under control. There was an exception, and that was when I went on a food binge. During all binges, I was alone.

I'm not sure why it is so important to eat food or drink at a gathering, or why people make other people feel so uncomfortable or embarrassed because he or she doesn't want to eat. People have their own reasons why, and that should be good enough. Much later on in my life, I learned this to be true of many situations. As a person who likes to control, I often questioned why people do what they do or don't do.

I have to keep telling myself it is none of my business how other people live. I guess I feel I am helping people with my advice or suggestions, hoping to make life easier for them. The thing is, it isn't up to me. People have to find their own happiness. That was what I did many years ago: looked for my happiness.

After graduation, in 1967, I traveled throughout Europe from October to December. The summer before, I worked as a lifeguard, swimming instructor, and playground advisor at a local pool to save a little money; but the main expense of the trip was a graduation gift from my parents.

While in Europe, I coped with the temperatures but found myself binging on fattening foods. I slowly entered a period where I wanted to eat all the time. The more I ate, the more weight I gained, and the more I wanted to eat. I became somewhat depressed, even though I was in beautiful surroundings. I fell prey to an unrecognizable lifestyle. I wasn't the person I wanted to be. I didn't like myself at all. My eating habits in high school were fine. What happened to change that in college? And now, what was so different in Europe to double the difficulty?

I thought a short haircut might change my state of mind. It felt great the first day. Then the *new feeling* quickly faded into the background. The real issue was still there. When I was alone, I was very unsettled and found myself looking for *something* to make it all better. My mind was scattered and confused. I didn't know why I continued to have so much trouble with food and being too warm after a meal. This problem went on long enough. There had to be an answer; however, each time I thought about it, my mind went blank.

My vacation ended, and I was back in Copake, living with my parents. I had no plans for the future. My high school and college days were over, and I felt the tension mounting. I had nothing in mind as far as what I wanted to do with my life or where I was going to live.

From whatever age we start remembering, from that point until I was nineteen, I idolized my parents and all their qualities. I desperately tried to be just like them, so much so I wasn't myself. I was so focused on wanting what they had and complaining about what I didn't, that I began to slip through the cracks.

As I looked at them each day, I envied the fact they were so grounded and comfortable in their own skin. They appeared to be content. I assumed they were happy with their lives. Why couldn't my life be happy?

While in Europe, I came in contact with many, different people who had diversified views on life. I started to form my own opinions, based on their influence. I wasn't sure if that was how I felt, but it seemed to make sense, especially for one who is looking for a perfect future.

The European people who crossed my path gave the impression of being very creative, free-spirited thinkers with fewer boundaries. Life seemed casual and relaxed. Deciding on your destiny wasn't that urgent at a young age. The message I received was to enjoy your youth, take your time in deciding, coast along for a while, and explore a little of the world. They enjoyed attention-grabbing conversations — ones that lasted for hours — and time was irrelevant.

Some of the people I met liked to discuss topics in great detail and then analyze what was said, similar to a debate. They learned from each other instead of arguing. When surrounded by this atmosphere, it was intoxicating, and it made my brain thirst for more. This was a whole new outlook, and it gave me something else to think about other than myself. I liked it, but it wasn't what I knew while growing up. At this age, it was easier to live life in a more Bohemian way, yet I knew when I returned home, a casual lifestyle wouldn't set well with my parents.

My parents sent me off to Europe upon my request. I had all the good reasons for going. I wanted to see the world, and it was a pleasurable trip. Truthfully, I think I went to escape the decision of where I was going with my life. It was adventuresome at the time and a good experience. I will be forever grateful for the gift. But when I came back, I still didn't have any answers.

I was eager to share my new enthusiasm though; however, it wasn't meant for the dinner table. In the time I was gone, I changed, and home was different, compared to when I was in high school. Something was off, and I wasn't sure what it was. I matured, so I thought. After all, I was a world traveler now. I was bubbly because I had a great deal to talk about, especially my new visions. However, once we were gathered around the table, I felt uneasy, as if I didn't fit in anymore.

My parents always enjoyed cocktail hour. That was nothing new. I believe it was the thing to do during the '50s in many households. Sometimes I felt it lasted a little longer than usual, which resulted in tense conversation that carried a negative energy. When I was younger I never noticed; now I sensed what was coming before it even happened.

I probably put too much emphasis on my feelings and, because I did, I suffered. I was very sensitive to what was discussed. Anything with a negative overtone sent me reeling. Unfortunately, I attempted to participate. Keeping silent would have been a better approach. We didn't agree on some topics, and those topics should have been left alone. And my new way of thinking didn't help.

The more I talked, the deeper I dug my hole. I presented my new outlook. I wasn't prepared for all the questions thrown my way, and I wanted to run back to my European friends. My answers weren't valid, and I didn't have enough information to substantiate what I said. I knew in my head how I wanted it to sound, but the words didn't come out right. Consequently, the discussion turned into an argument.

During these moments, I felt the blood rush to my head. Once it began, there was no stopping it. My neck became tight with tension, as if someone wrapped a rubber band around it. I swallowed extra air, hoping to calm myself down, and, before I knew it, the frustration and upset ruined my appetite for dinner. I didn't have my new friends there to help explain my thoughts. When all was said and done, I was pretty much convinced my life would never be what it once was.

I grew up with the idea that I was supposed to select an occupation before I graduated from high school and, once I had a degree, go to work.

The thing is, each person's makeup is different. Some take longer than others to decide. Medical conditions can interfere with his or her choices. Some people learn faster and more easily than others. I don't believe there is a cookie-cutter mold for each of us.

Situations and people can cross our paths, and our destinies change. People have to work their way through to what is right for them. Maybe we fail; maybe we luck out. I believe that as long as we are still breathing, we have a chance. When we are young, there is so much thrown at us, and, truly, it can be very difficult and confusing.

When any unhappy topic was discussed at the dinner table, I withdrew. My ears turned red, so much so, I couldn't eat. My mind and body wanted to flee. Mealtime was where I was most vulnerable. I compensated my ignorance by being arrogant and didn't realize I was putting a block between us. I tried to keep a conversation going so we didn't sit in silence. I got so I dreaded mealtime.

Dad and I drifted apart, and I didn't feel as close to either of my parents as I once did, which was sad. I also felt I was the guilty party for causing this separation.

I was the one who had the problem. I allowed words and emotions to affect my appetite, and, unfortunately, the loss of appetite didn't stop with one meal. I was not mature enough to handle the unpleasant moments, and every time I sat down to a meal, I was on guard, waiting for a negative conversation to begin. This became a lifelong issue.

While in high school, I flew to Colorado and stayed with one of Dad's army buddies and his family. As the plane soared into the air and floated among the clouds, I felt as if I were in heaven. Then I noticed how peaceful, clean, and orderly everything was. Compared to life on the ground, the atmosphere in the cabin was less chaotic. Everything and everyone had a place. The attendants didn't have to decide what to wear each day; the uniform made each one equally beautiful in appearance. As soon as a passenger needed the least amount of assistance, a stewardess was present. I found this to be true each time I flew. The whole scene brought me to a place where I wanted to be.

The idea of finding a job escalated, and then I remembered this experience and thought maybe a career as an airline stewardess was an option. I was sure my parents would be happy with my choice. Again, my need for approval surfaced. I wanted so much to fit into society, and I was happy about finally making a decision.

On the day of the interview, I was very nervous, a normal trait for me when I was *under fire*. I just squeaked through on the height requirement. I squeezed my wrist just for something to do and felt my pulse pounding. That meant my heart was racing a mile a minute, and I anticipated the end of the interview before it even began. I just wanted it to be over. When I left the office, I couldn't remember anything the interviewer said, it was all a blur. The day the letter arrived from the airline, I think I knew the answer before I opened it. I wasn't accepted.

If I evaluated what I did well, that left a career in swimming or cooking. Ironically, both are connected to either water or food.

I finally decided to get a job locally. I went to work for a large, gift house in Great Barrington, Massachusetts, but I left after a couple of months.

None of my jobs lasted. Wherever I worked, my employment only lasted from one to three months. The first day was always exciting, and I was pumped. As soon as I went on lunch break, the heat monster from the past appeared. Overwhelmed with stress about managing a meal at work, then attempting to work as if I were going through menopause, I usually ended up quitting.

Job after job, after job, my heat problem never got better. In every lunchroom, it was as if someone played tricks on me and deliberately turned up the heat as soon as I entered, and then kept laughing at me while I suffered.

I knew I had to work somewhere, so I kept trying, always hoping my problem would change for the better. I even developed a phobia about eating with co-workers. I thought if I ate alone maybe I could control the elements through psychic powers. A few times, I thought it worked, but I could never count on it. I concluded it just happened that way by chance.

Normal drifted away. Food choice, and my environment, either destroyed the day or made it okay. Some of the side effects were not only uncomfortable but also embarrassing. When my face and ears turned red, and it lasted longer and longer, I tried to hide it with my hands or by turning my head so people couldn't see what I was feeling. The warmth in my head was a distraction from my job performance. What to eat and what to wear was a *depressing, daily challenge*. I became less interested in eating. The task wasn't the problem; it was the struggle of *choice*. I never knew what the outcome was going to be. Each morning, as I dressed for work, I wondered how long I would last before I became so hot that I wanted to remove all my clothes. That is why I often wore the same outfit many days in a row. If by chance I tolerated the material, the relief was worth it.

When I was in college, I sent away for a five-dollar, denim skirt. The first time I put it on, I knew it was perfect. The material felt magnificent next to my skin, no matter how long I wore the skirt. In fact, I wore it just about every day in college. I continued wearing it throughout the summer, much to my mother's dismay. The skirt became raggedy and worn out, but I wouldn't give it up. I didn't realize at the time what I was doing. It didn't even dawn on me that I was creating an obsession. When I dressed in this denim skirt, I felt normal. That was all I asked for. I wanted my skin to feel normal, and most of the time, it didn't. At times, the heat I felt throughout my body was so intense, all my thinking wrapped around that one thought.

When the heat became unbearable at work, I compensated by moving around constantly, wishing that would help. I probably made more trips to the restroom than any other employee.

Often, I would sneak outside to cool off, only to return much warmer than before I went out. This procedure only upset me more. When I did eat, I chose the wrong foods. I had good intentions, but when I dined with other people, my taste buds weren't satisfied. The next thing I knew, I was *alone*, looking for a cold spot. When I was cold, and *alone*, my appetite increased so much that I ended up overeating. Consequently, the bathroom scale read much higher than I preferred.

My stress level escalated when I thought about going to work. I couldn't sleep, my nutrition was poor, and I was *depressed*. I did not know what was wrong. Nothing changed for the better. I was sure no one would understand, and besides, I didn't know how to explain what I was feeling without making it sound psychological, so I kept all my emotions inside. Soon *all* job prospects looked grim.

I expected my adult life to be as *normal*, but my picture had a missing piece. My health changed; I didn't know what it was, but I knew it wasn't right. I had surges of heat that didn't allow me to sit still. I craved foods I didn't want to eat, and the more I tried to eat sensibly, the more I ate insensibly. I was scared. It was time to make my way and leave home, and I felt helpless and hopeless. The days were never-ending as the winter dragged on.

The spring of 1968 arrived, and I was temporarily happy once again. My parents told me I could stay at our cabin at Copake Lake for the summer. That was good news, because I could swim every day to my heart's desire.

The stress I felt lessened. Every morning, the lake's beauty greeted me. It only took a few steps, and I was caressed by its coolness. For now, life couldn't get any better.

Chapter 3
You Never Know

It was 1968 when I decided to contact an old college roommate, and I invited her to spend a weekend with me at our cabin on Copake Lake. We talked about all the things young women talk about. I complained about my weight gain. I was disgusted and ashamed that I gained so much weight. She suggested a diet that worked well for her. It sounded good, and also healthy.

My friend worked in New York City at one of the top magazines. All day long, she came in contact with the world of fashion. When we discussed the difficulties I had in finding employment and my short-term involvement in the workforce, she mentioned there was a good chance she could help me find a job in the city.

I knew I had to find work. Never in my wildest dreams did I think I might be working in New York City. I was there on a short-term basis for my college internship, but this was different. A new spark of enthusiasm materialized in my brain. One thought led to another thought, and before I knew it, I pictured this new concept working for me. This could really become my future home. My heat problem still existed, but the more my friend and I talked, I believed the city was my answer to a new life. At first, the urgency to find work was to satisfy the people who loved me. After hearing about this new adventure, I was ready to move right away.

I continued discussing what was going on in my life, and I confessed my obsession for walking and why it was so important to me. I said I felt stagnant and trapped in a small town. I was going nowhere, and walking gave me the illusion of going somewhere. The idea of having to walk every day gave my life meaning. It was an accomplishment I looked forward to. That discussion was the closest I came to revealing my problems to anyone.

The frequent interludes of excessive heat, especially my head at mealtime or when I was indoors for any length of time, were often eliminated, briefly, after a nice long walk. Walking became an escape. It seemed to relieve the pain. It gave me the feeling of coolness as long as I kept moving. This is where habitual walking became very important.

My friend believed a change of scenery would be a good place to start, plus New York City had unlimited walking areas. From my viewpoint, summer was coming, and there would be air-conditioning in the buildings to help with my overheated body, especially my head. I was totally ecstatic of the picture she drew of city life.

She contacted the McCall's Pattern Company and arranged an interview. She also found me a residence for women. It all sounded too good to be true. I went to the interview and was hired shortly after.

As the train pulled into Grand Central Station, my adrenaline was up. My heart gained an extra beat when I thought of what lie ahead. I was nervous but excited. This was big. Being on my own in one of the largest cities was an amazing feeling. I had an incredible sensation of freedom, like anything was possible. To top it off, I had the job at McCall's. I was sure this was a turning point to a better life. I was going to make it this time! I just knew it!

I walked through the last door of the station and out onto the busy street. There was so much space for my feet to travel. I was in heaven, with the endless array of streets calling out to me. I knew, at this moment, I would be walking to every destination. And that was a good thing.

When I arrived in this glorious kingdom, it was a warm, July day, and the heat pushed its way upward from the pavement. The residence for girls was only a short distance from the station, so it seemed rather sensible to walk. With every step I took, I brought extra air into my lungs, hoping to alleviate the overwhelming heat. My feelings of discomfort were negated by my enthusiasm, and I believed that in time I would get used to it. After all, this was only the first day.

The residence was operated by the Catholic Church and, thankfully, in a safe neighborhood. The price was certainly reasonable, only twenty-seven dollars a month, which included two meals, linens, and a comfortable lounge on the ground floor. By the time I lugged several, heavy suitcases from Grand Central, through the Pan American Building, across another avenue, and then finally arrived on Third Avenue, I was hot and tired. There obviously wasn't a nice, cool lake to jump into — as it turned out, only a hot, old building with no air conditioning. My room was up three flights of stairs and was the size of a small closet. But as I sat on the bed and gazed around the room, I was happy with my new home. It was quaint, and I loved it, even though it was down to the bare essentials: a bed and mattress, a miniature sink hanging from the wall, a simple chair, and tiny closet. This was a symbol of my life at the moment. The room and I were stripped and starting over.

The bed was without sheets, and each renter became her own maid. I walked up to the top floor for linens, and this day was a sizzler, so by that time, I was wringing wet with perspiration. I definitely needed a shower, and, thank God, it was on my floor. After freshening up, I dressed for dinner and was on my way to settle in.

As I walked into the dining room, my appetite faded. The heat of the room surrounded me, and I felt as if I couldn't breathe. I had just changed into a nice, cool, summer dress; but as I stood at the entrance, it felt more like I was wearing a wool jumpsuit. A huge fan at the far end of the eating area did nothing to cool the room or me. The chef served meatloaf and mashed potatoes — not something one generally eats on a scorching hot day. There was no way I would eat there. I did a complete turn around and headed for the exit door. From then on, I knew lunch and dinner would be eaten in an air-conditioned restaurant.

The diet, my friend and I discussed, started immediately. An essential part of the diet was to eat, at least, five meals of fish each week. As I walked out of the residence, my eyes searched for a seafood sign. Not even a block away, was a great, seafood restaurant with air-conditioning. It was *perfect*.

After a long relaxing dinner in very cool surroundings, I walked several blocks, taking in all the sights and smells of the city. For a country gal, this was quite something. It was hard to believe I was actually walking the streets of New York City everyday. After spending time in a very cool environment, I was able to briefly tolerate the outdoor heat. In many ways, my life became a pattern of inconsistencies. I hated the heat in general; however, outdoor heat was more manageable than indoor heat. I believe the reasoning behind this was movement. Whenever I was outdoors I was in motion. I avoided standing still or sitting.

That first day, and for the rest of the summer, every step I took boosted my spirits. I walked to work, walked to lunch, walked home, walked to dinner, and walked after dinner. Anyone else would have recognized I had developed a compulsion to walk. I couldn't go to sleep without an evening walk. Occasionally, I was tired and didn't feel like walking. However, I felt guilty if I didn't walk every day, and my evening stroll had to last a certain amount of time. The pattern developed.

My sister came to visit for a weekend and brought a girlfriend with her. Before the first night was over, I made sure we went for a walk! I was used to walking, and I didn't think anything of it as I had them follow me up and down the avenues. They were totally exhausted by the time the weekend was over.

Every morning upon rising, I did a set of exercises, even in a very warm room. I tried not to think about the heat. Again, I felt guilty if I didn't complete the routine every day.

Then I quickly dressed and made my way to the very warm dining hall. I managed breakfast at the residence, because I didn't want to start my day by looking for a restaurant and then finding it more uncomfortable than what was in front of me. And I wasn't in the residence that long before I was on my way to an air-conditioned office. I ate a quick, simple breakfast, with very little fat and no sugar. I alternated a poached egg and dry, wheat toast, juice, and black coffee with a breakfast of dry, wheat toast and a slice of low-calorie cheese, juice, and black coffee. No matter how inviting the cafeteria food looked, I stuck with the same items — never wavering. Many years later, I realized this healthy diet was probably lessening the heat in the body, along with walking and losing weight.

There was a well-used refrigerator in the basement of the residence, and renters were allowed to store a few items in it. Cheese was part of my skimpy, breakfast diet and couldn't be left in my room. When I first laid eyes on this old, worn-out icebox, it seemed to be the perfect solution, but I wondered if it kept anything cold. It worked fine; however, more times than not, my cheese disappeared. I even placed the package in different areas or behind an item in the refrigerator to make it more difficult for my thief. Still, the entire package of cheese vanished from time to time.

I became very emotional and angry, and then questioned *why*. Why would anyone steal someone else's food? I never experienced anything like this before. I had most of my day under control: a good night sleep, morning exercise, dress, eat, and walk to work. I liked the routine, and my confidence improved. But when someone pulled a prank like stealing my food, I didn't think it was funny. I planned out every part of the morning like clockwork. Something like this was not supposed to happen. As I stared into the refrigerator with disbelief, my nerves got the best of me. I wanted to shout at someone, but whom? I didn't have any idea who the thief was.

Then I panicked. I had to be at work. I didn't have the luxury of wasting time. However, I would not substitute another food for the cheese, not even for one day. I had to have cheese. It was part of the pattern that made my day work. It was in the new diet, which helped me lose weight. With very little time to spare before work, I frantically left the building to look for cheese. Luckily, a deli wasn't too far away.

I returned to the residence, quickly ate, and rushed to work. The problem was fixed, but only for a day. And it was quite inconvenient. From then on, I was never sure if my cheese would be available when I needed it.

There was a coffee shop that offered just what I wanted for my luncheon meal. It was located just below the office, so I had ample time to eat. And I had a favorite table. The cool air poured straight down on my head and gave me a terrific appetite. Each day, as I entered the coffee shop, I held my breath in hopes my table would be vacant. As soon as I entered the eatery, I rushed past customers and *grabbed it* before someone else sat down — as if I were playing musical chairs.

After dinner, I went with a friend to a nearby, air-conditioned deli until it was time for bed. We had the most interesting discussions while slowly sipping our coffee. Most evenings, we sat for hours soaking up the atmosphere and allowing ourselves to drift into the perfect surroundings. These moments became very special. The world outside didn't exist. Everything I needed was right in front of me: a perfect temperature and companionship.

Occasionally, my friend suggested going to another restaurant. I feared a new location and was insistent on only meeting at the same spot. Not realizing it at the time, I wanted control of the situation. Yet I wanted friends. The time we met was on my terms. Most evenings, it worked out for both of us. If she had plans, I became depressed. My normal routine was altered.

Against my better judgment, I gave in to a blind date she planned. I had one stipulation: we had to walk to the restaurant.

The eatery was on the other side of town. And to add more misery and stress, I was concerned about the menu. My daily meals were well planned before each day. I knew where and what I would be eating. This was a new restaurant I knew nothing about. I was also concerned with weight gain; therefore, I insisted we walk back home afterwards. The evening was tense. I pretended to have a good time. However, I wanted to be at my usual restaurant in the neighborhood near the residence instead. I never saw my date again.

The main part of my job was to set up a lecture schedule for a group of girls. They traveled the country, promoting McCall's Patterns. When they came back to the city, they put together their new, clothing line for the following season. I was also in charge of scheduling their entertainment, usually a Broadway show. The job at McCall's was a very positive, and much-needed, element in my life. I liked having a structured day and doing the same thing daily. This made me feel secure and confident.

The most difficult part of my job was sitting in an office all day long. I grew restless, and, from time to time, I took walks to the restroom just to move around. Then I delayed my return by chatting with a fellow worker about work-related issues. I purposely talked about work, so I wouldn't get fired. But my behavior was noticed, and I was summoned to the boss's office several times on both matters.

Each workday, I looked forward to the weekend. It meant I could walk all I wanted and not be stuck at a desk, but when Friday night arrived, ironically, I felt lost. To fill in the empty time, I returned to my hometown of Copake. Two days were spent on the train, which only left one day of forlorn emptiness. On Sunday evening, my mother drove me to the small, but quaint, train station in Copake Falls. The station was closed for years, and the whole area looked rather sad in my eyes.

I often scanned the building, saw its possibilities, and said to my mother, "I wish someone would take over the station and fix it up. If I had my way, the station would be just like it was in the good ol' days." More times than not, I believe what I really wanted was to live in the past.

Each Sunday night, as I boarded the train, I felt a rush of excitement; I was on my way back to the beautiful city. I eagerly walked to my seat and settled in with good book and a Delicious apple. There was always a special place in my heart for New York City, and the thrill of coming into Grand Central Station never grew old. I loved every train ride that brought me back to this amazing city, and now it was my new home. I visited there many times when I was younger, but now it was different. I was on my own, and I had a job. I also enjoyed the hustle and bustle, the fast pace, and even the noise; all were comforting.

When I moved to the city, I weighed 160 pounds. The more weight I lost, the cooler I felt. I was able to endure more heat as long as I stuck to my diet. Even so, I continued to look for *very cold* air-conditioning for lunch and dinner.

Ironically, I tolerated only a fan at night when I went to sleep, and I slept terrific. Back home, in the still of the night, I tossed and turned, and tortured myself with negative thoughts — complaining of the heat, or being awakened by a creak in the floorboard or from a raccoon near my window eating leftovers in the garbage pail. Why was it so different here? I believe it was a combination of things. First of all, I was happy. My days were full, and every evening, as I walked along the avenue, I stripped everything from my mind and enjoyed the moment. When I put my head on the pillow, I was at peace. The warm, evening air was relaxing, and with the fan on, before I knew it, I was asleep like a baby. Not even a fire alarm, sirens, or fights in the street were disruptive.

My weight reduction program was going well, except for the seventh day of the week when I craved everything that wasn't on the diet: spicy, salty, fatty, and creamy! I was losing a considerable amount of weight, and maybe my body was telling me that I was starving myself of the items I had completely eliminated — like a little fat now and then. I needed a variety of foods, in moderation, but I didn't pay attention to the signs. On the last day of the week, I *binged*.

I went to what I called my favorite Italian, *binge* restaurant. They had the best flavorful, Italian dishes, excellent ice cream, and cheesecake that took me back to the days I spent in Italy. Normally, I did not drink alcohol or eat sweets, but on *binge* night, that changed. I craved everything fattening, and the alcohol induced my appetite even more.

When I left the restaurant, I stopped for more ice cream at another establishment and, at another shop, for more cheesecake. After that, I walked a little farther to a grocery store for ice cream and a candy bar. The ice cream only cooled me down temporarily. As soon as it was digested, I was so warm I had to keep walking. If I sat down, the heat rushed to my head, and I felt sick.

I continued this destructive pattern until I couldn't eat one more morsel of food. I felt like junk. I took a laxative before I went to bed for several reasons: to dispose of the food that was now setting my body on fire, to take away any weight I gained, and to rid my mind of the guilt. I had given in to heavy caloric foods that would put the lost weight back on.

The air-conditioning, eating very low-energy foods, and losing weight all could have lowered my body temperature. This wasn't on my mind at the time. I was sufficiently *warm as I slept* but not miserably hot. During the day, I avoided my small room, as the heat there rose to almost inhumane conditions. I was able to withstand *walking in the heat* when there was a gentle breeze. I found it relaxing and cooling. I *binged* on the seventh day of the week. These three things probably worked like a blanket of protection, keeping my temperature stable. I didn't understand any of this until much later in life.

Although a new problem — my weekly binge — developed, I loved my new life in the city. Walking to all my destinations actually gave me a spectacular high, as if I were Mary Poppins, with an umbrella in my hand, floating over the rooftops. I also liked the freedom of the limitless city. It made my skin feel good, the same skin that frequently made me feel trapped and uncomfortable. Whenever I was out walking, I was not window-shopping and never stopped to buy clothes.

I walked solely to walk. Taking a walk on a warm, summer's evening, with the soft air caressing my body, was more than perfect. It was the most peaceful way to end the day.

I felt as if my whole life had meaning. I was a woman of the business world, and I had a handle on my life. My new routine in my new surroundings, plus the weight loss, made me believe I had the heat problem and the weight problem under control. Whether I was in the city, or back home in the country, I held my head high and carried an imaginary sign that read, "I've got it together." I was finally content.

The summer at McCall's was wonderful for me, but it flew by too quickly, and the cooler days of autumn arrived. The patterns I so carefully developed were disrupted, and my life was turned upside down once again. The air-conditioning went off in the buildings, and the heat came on.

I felt as if I were on fire as the heat engulfed me. The usual workday was a blur. I sat and stared at the paperwork, and nothing was accomplished. No matter how hard I tried to concentrate, nothing mattered any more. The temperatures were reversed. I couldn't take being indoors, and walking outdoors was very uncomfortable in the cool air. I needed warm air against my skin when outdoors and cool air when I came indoors. I complained to a friend, and she told me to put on a heavy coat and walk outdoors. All that did was make me too warm from the neck down, and when I returned indoors, I burned up from head to toe.

Everything I ate made me hot, as well as my clothing. Sitting in the lobby of the women's residence and staring into space, I asked myself what went wrong.

I called my father telling him of my problems, stating the interior of every building — commercial or otherwise — felt too warm for me to function. There was too much difficulty to eat, sleep, or work. Dreading meals, I ate very little, which made me feel sick to my stomach all the time, and contributed to lost days at work. He didn't have an answer to my dilemma.

Right from that first day, when I boarded the train in Copake Falls and headed to New York City, I was sure my life was going to change for the better and that anything was possible. The endless, depressing days of feeling like I was going nowhere would end. My overweight body would become trim. I could return home and be proud of my new life. That feeling of being hot all the time would be gone. Living in that wondrous city was going to solve all my problems. That's what I thought.

Instead, I had failed again. Instead of conquering my problems, they had intensified, and I had new behaviors that would have their own repercussions.

Chapter 4
The Light Went Out

I left the exciting city to what seemed to be the dull country. Everything that fell into place like a perfect sculpture was now smashed into a million pieces. When I went to New York City in the spring of 1968, I weighed 160 pounds. When I left, I weighed 110 pounds. I was more than happy for a couple of months. I lost a lot of weight, and, for once, I was comfortable with the size of my body and pleased with my appearance. At least, I accomplished that much. People commented that I looked like Twiggy; I didn't see it.

The lifestyle in the city was fast paced and colorful. Every day was structured with excitement. Even though I grew up in the country, coming back to it was not uplifting. I tried to make the best of it; however, all I thought about was how content I was in New York City. Now, that part of my life was gone.

Days went by, and I saw myself going downhill. I lost interest in everything. I had nothing to look forward to. I felt as though I failed. The internal heat I felt wasn't going away. Finally, after trying to cope for many months, I couldn't take it anymore. I had to fill the void with something stimulating. I decided to go south. I was going to recreate what I experienced in New York City.

I had some savings, and in 1969, during the St. Patrick's Day Parade in New York City, I boarded a train to Florida. I stayed with an elderly woman, who happened to be a friend of my grandparents. Florida wasn't New York City. The days were empty with no direction. And the diet I once followed wasn't working. The heat monster must have slipped into my suitcase because I soon found it difficult to function. My plan didn't work. I stayed three months before returning home. I was very unsettled. The confidence I had while living in the city was quickly slipping away.

My cousin often stopped in to visit, and with him came a ray of sunshine. When he appeared at the door I was happy. He brought with him a positive energy that awakened my spirit. Much of his visit was spent with my father watching sports on television. However, his company put a bounce in my step. It was as if someone woke me from a long sleep. At that point in my life, I yearned to have new life in the house. It seemed to be a diversion from my troubles. I still had to deal with my issues when I was alone, but for the moment, it was good.

Totally bored, and with nothing specific in mind, the days ahead looked bleak. I kept telling myself I had to do something even if it was wrong.

In January 1970, a girlfriend and I left for California, land of sun and fun. Prior to leaving, I noticed I was gaining too much weight so I asked my family doctor for diet pills. Wow, the energy I developed was astounding. I could have torn down a house and rebuilt it. The pills boosted my spirits and created a positive mood. Everything around me was beautiful until the pill wore off, then I was depressed. The day wasn't as colorful. All my issues came rushing back to haunt me.

The one thing I noticed right away was my ravenous appetite. I tried to ignore it and eat sparingly. I just couldn't. My body craved more food than ever. And then I yearned for another happy pill, even though they made my life unreal. These pills were supposed to be diet pills; instead, I gained weight. Giving up a euphoric high wasn't easy, but I finally stopped taking them.

I worked the night shift at the Grand Hotel coffee shop in Anaheim for three months. I soon realized the grass wasn't any greener on the West Coast, and I returned to the east coast in March 1970.

The secure, idyllic, fairytale life I had as a child and teenager was gone forever. Now, my life was open to choice, and I didn't have a clue where my future was headed. I was in a rut, wasting time. The more I thought about the perfect life I once had, the more upset I became. How would I ever make anything of myself and truly be happy as long as I had this beast of heat lurking in my body.

When I was young, my parents often spoke of the past and their memories. My mother's descriptions made it easy to picture the *olden days*. We often visited historical landmarks, which heightened my enthusiasm. I was fascinated with the estates of yesteryear, clothing from a different time period, and how people lived, in general. It seemed to me that life was simpler, and possibly more meaningful, when people had less. Maybe I didn't want to face my future. Possibly, I allowed my thoughts to escape into another age, as if it were a make believe movie that I was apart of.

The reality of being an adult and leaving the nest was not a good subject. I tried to ignore it and hold on to the safe feeling. I was overly sensitive and felt the tension in the air; I was certainly in a screwed up situation. I believe my parents saw an unhappy child, one who wasn't progressing or moving on in her life. My lifestyle probably came across as a mental problem. Either way, there wasn't a simple explanation.

From then on, my days went from bad to worse. I felt as if I had to keep moving every waking hour. I had no self-assurance. I was in turmoil, mentally, not knowing what was happening to my life. I didn't want to sit and talk to anyone about any of this. I was ill at ease with my lifestyle and waited for disapproval from anyone who wanted to give it, which was no one. I felt it though. I was sure there was dissatisfaction written all over onlookers' faces. Each day was a huge void with no progress. A vast nothingness continued on and on with no end in sight.

Physically, I was challenged because I wanted to be forever cool. No matter what I did with my body, I overheated. I got to a point where I put off meals as long as I could. People around me were enjoying food; I made up excuses and said I wasn't hungry. Then I wanted to eat alone. I did get that wish. I was alone in many ways.

I tried working at a hospital in Albany, New York, which lasted all of three months. I returned home and, in 1970, opened my own small, gift shop. Because of my major in college, I thought maybe this might be the answer to my *going-nowhere* existence. I believed by returning home, all my problems would be solved. An unrealistic projection, but one I desperately wanted to be true: all my distress would go away. Again, I thought I had a plan.

I christened the store Dandy Lion Boutique. Preparing for opening day was hectic, but it kept my mind occupied and my body busy. As long as I had a long *to do list*, I ran on a false energy, and I loved it. I painted the side of an adjacent building with bugs and butterflies. Then I designed and painted an animated sign to coincide with my store's name. My neighbor helped out with display cases, and my mother pitched in wherever she was needed.

Eating in the store was not an option. I put up a mental block and convinced myself I couldn't dine there. When it came time for a meal, I closed up the shop and headed home. Each day, I prayed no one would be in the kitchen when I walked through the door. An unrealistic notion, but one I clung to. Of course, that rarely happened. Why I needed this existence was never clear to me. I pretended it didn't matter; however, all along, my emotions were on overdrive and my nutrition suffered.

The first week was all a *buzz*. Children from the local camps loved the penny candy. It actually paid the monthly rent. Business was very upbeat for about two weeks. After that, everything changed. I had very few customers, plus all the *hands-on work* was done.

Sitting alone in the store, I felt trapped and overwhelmed with heat. I attempted to evaluate my situation. I saw a pattern in all of this: as long as I had something to do, where I moved around, the heat wasn't so bad. Of course, we all have to sit still occasionally; the body can't be in motion all the time.

Whenever I was able to escape from the store, I went to our cabin at the lake and took a quick swim. Each time, I stayed a little longer. Occasionally, my mother or father went to the store. If I returned late, I was questioned as to my whereabouts, along with an unapproved look. They had no clue what was going on with my body. I didn't explain it either.

Sitting in the store became almost unbearable. I paced around the shop in circles. My neighbor made a loom, and I wove belts to pass the time. The heat I felt consumed every part of me. I thought I would go out of my mind with anxiety. Fear became an obsession. The grave anticipation of each workday tore at my soul.

It wasn't long before I closed up the shop and fled to the lake. As I drove down the dirt road to the cabin, I felt the freedom. All the car windows were open, and the wind swished and swirled around my head like a windstorm. In only a few minutes, I would be stripped of my clothes and drenched in cool water. While sitting in the shop each day, I reminisced this interlude. Before I knew it, the water was my driving force to stay alive.

Winter arrived, and the Dandy Lion Boutique had very little business. I decided to lock the door for several months. In 1971, my cousin and I drove to Colorado Springs, where my sister was attending college.

Once we were settled, there was nothing to do except look forward to meals. Everyone else had a life.

I was even very rude to my cousin. There was a possibility she could live elsewhere, and I almost insisted she leave the apartment we were staying in. I wanted to be alone. I didn't explain why. I was too embarrassed to say I wanted to eat my meals with no one else around. I was afraid of becoming too hot.

Eventually, the day became an empty hole; I became restless. I don't know why I wanted to return to Copake. I wasn't content there either. At this point in time, there were no other options, plus I was running out of money. It wasn't long before we *hit* the road and headed back east.

When I arrived home, even though I still had my own store, I worked for a couple of months in the neighboring town for two of my friends. The atmosphere was enchanting and elegant; however, the days were long as I waited for customers.

There was an apartment over the store, and that is where I ate lunch. This part of the day was still a thorn and something I didn't take pleasure in. On most days, the store was chilly. That factor gave me the *go ahead* for consuming a high fat food. The store carried homemade peanut butter and oven-baked bread. I thought about these two items all morning. I prayed for cool surroundings, void of people. It never failed; as soon as I began eating, someone walked up the stairs and entered the same room I was in. The presence of another body created heat.

I used to torment myself by wishing I could control the atmosphere around me. But this didn't work either. As soon as I entered a warm room, all the heat rushed back into my body. It was useless. I had to eat something, so I forced the food down. The heat crept up my spine and consumed my body like a fire taking over a building. In my mind, the day was ruined. My only hope to cool off came from the coolers in the cellar. A catalog was placed on the counter with each frozen food listed, along with the price. Eagerly, I waited for customers in need of those items.

Trips to the cellar and watching the clock were popular pastimes. Between focusing on the minutes, and hiding out in the cellar, I didn't think the day would ever end.

The owners involved me in one of their New York buying trips, which included a dinner at a rather fancy restaurant. As we entered the eatery, I didn't know how I would manage to eat a full dinner in unfamiliar surroundings and impress two men who didn't have any idea what my secret life was all about. And I didn't want them to know. I ordered two beers, and my appetite improved significantly. Regrettably, I couldn't stop eating, and I even swiped all the dinner mints from the table to devour on the ride back to Copake. I arrived home very late and continued to binge before bed. Then the betrayal set in. I messed up my body by gorging and stuffing so much food into my system. Why?

From the outside, I looked perfectly normal with no issues at all. For years and years, I hid what was happening on the inside. I put on a smiley face when I was with people, but alone, I was sad. I made believe my life was fine. This wasn't the case. Every day became more difficult and gloomier. I was nervous about eating every meal. I wished I didn't have to eat, or there was a pill that took the place of food. An hour or two after a meal, I seemed to adjust, and my skin began to feel normal. Then it was time to eat again. I felt as if I were a mouse running on a treadmill and getting nowhere.

The Dandy Lion Boutique was open for a little over a year and a half. Business was slow, and I was in an unsettling condition. As the warm weather approached, in the spring of 1972, I spent less time there. It only took me ten minutes to drive to my peaceful retreat, Copake Lake. It was only natural for me to gravitate back to my paradise when I was in such turmoil. I left the store several times a day to douse myself in the cool waters and extinguish the heat I felt. It was a temporary cool. Once I came out of the water, my skin was hot again. Any activity — for example, a short walk — heated me up. It was easy to conclude I needed cool water throughout the day, no matter what I did. I found myself back in the cool water more times than I realized.

From 1972 to 1975 I swam in cold water, at least, four times a day.
And I took a cold shower four times a day.

My father set up charge accounts at various grocery stores and a gas station. Whenever I needed food or gas, I was able to charge it, and my father paid those bills each month. I was very fortunate in that respect. Occasionally, I worked in my father's office at the funeral home, doing some bookkeeping. Once in a while, he asked me to take *calling hours*. I never wanted to leave the lake and the cold water; however, I felt some obligation, because they were paying all my expenses. The cold water felt good on my skin, but the air-conditioning didn't supply the same relief.

I dreaded going into town for groceries. It appeared to be a long, hot drive because the farther I was from the lake, the less control I had over my life. As the distance grew the heat escalated. The only asset was the storeowner. He never questioned my actions. He treated me with kindness and respect. He saw my attire, the look on my face, the uneasiness of my character, and for the time being — a going nowhere — existence. He knew I hid away at the lake because of something, but didn't question as to why. Maybe he felt it was my responsibility to find myself and live that life. Because, whoever I was, someday that period of my survival would be my gift back to the world; individualism is highly honored by some folks.

Soon, the swimming wasn't enough to cool me off, and I began taking cold showers. That didn't sustain me either. While I was still wet from the shower, I sat in front of a fan and ate my meals — a ritual that was quickly adopted and not easily destroyed. No one knew of this behavior; I wanted it kept secret. The routine felt strange, even to me, and I was ashamed. I certainly didn't want my parents to know.

I was alone in the cabin for the summer, but sometimes my mother stopped in unannounced. I didn't want her to see what I was doing. So I nervously pretended I was busy and didn't have time to spend with her. I knew she was hurt by my aloofness that summer. I didn't want to upset her by acting disinterested in her visit, but I didn't know how to explain to my own mother that this overheated body I was living in controlled my life, and I couldn't stop it.

I was at a point in my life where I forced myself to swim, even when I didn't want to, prior to every meal. I looked for very cool water. If it was cold, that was even better. I was so worn out that meals lost their appeal, and they weren't satisfying.

After finishing a meal, I still had cravings. I satisfied them with ice cream at first. I consumed, at least, a pint of ice cream, several cookies, and then candy. The heavy sweetness made me feel sick, so I ate bread with lots of butter, then back to the ice cream, and more sweets. The *binge* foods slid down effortlessly. Shortly afterward, I felt terrible. While I ate those tasty treats, I wasn't hot; but once they started to metabolize, my body felt as if I was caged in a hot box with no air. I also gained weight, which was *depressing*.

With all the down moments, I *never* thought about suicide. Life was too precious. I wanted to live at any cost. Somehow I would make it.

I was still living at home, whether it was at the cabin or with Mom and Dad. I just didn't fit in any place, in my body, or in my parents' house. My life was not on track.

In the winter months, the obvious substitute for the cold, lake water would be a cold shower, but that wasn't a fix for the heat I felt; I had to be exercising extensively while in the cold water. The winter was a nightmare. I depended on the lake to take the fire out of my skin, but I couldn't swim in the lake with a layer of ice on it. During the winter, the heat I felt was more intense than in the summer. I was suffering and going nowhere. I did not know how to explain to myself the mess I was in, let alone fix it.

Chapter 5
The Divine Feeling of Water

The medical definition of addiction is a physical dependence on a drug or some other substance that is ingested or inhaled in some form that causes an alteration in brain functioning and depends on the substance for normal functioning. Examples are drug addiction and alcoholism.

My definition is a little different, but then so is my perspective. I look at addiction from the inside out.

I define addiction as when a substance or an action takes over a person's life to a point where he or she feels a compulsive need to continue it regularly in order to function and survive. I emphasize regularly. An individual *may* have a choice when the circumstances first occur, before the urge becomes a need or requirement. Eventually, the individual will do anything in his or her power to continue this obsessive *thing*. The addiction totally interferes with daily life. People who are addicted have no life. Their life becomes an attempt to fulfill the compulsion.

I believe addictions go further than the medical definition. I question why the substance has to be a drug. Why can't it be the inhalation of cold air, or submersion into cold water, or ingestion of cold liquids and cold food in a very cold environment? This will definitely cause an alteration in the brain.

I engulfed my body in excessive, cold temperatures for months. The result for me was a body temperature of eighty-eight degrees. When ice was taken away from me, I stopped eating for forty days. And without this cold, I believed I was nothing.

While I struggled with my addiction, I barely functioned. I withdrew from society. I could not work, or eat, or sleep without being in cold water. It was the single most important thing in my life for sixteen years.

If someone questions whether I was addicted or not, in my mind, I will always believe that I was addicted to cold water.

Swimming was a big part of my life. People often said, "Jill would rather be in the water than out."

I felt comfortable in the water, as if it were my natural habitat. The feel of water around me — the coolness — was soothing. It caressed my body and made me feel whole. I was at peace.

At this time in my life, when I was in such distress, I reached back into my past. Swimming appeared to be the answer to the agony I felt. For the first time in years, I was somewhat relieved.

I never expected an enjoyable sport to become an addiction. I didn't foresee any harm in something so beneficial. It was an excuse to get out of the house and maybe meet new people; it was something to look forward to, and a place to go. My mental and physical state would be fulfilled. There was no doubt in my mind. I was going to swim every day.

I was bored with the daily routine at the lake. I had shut everyone out. I was lonely. Other than the swimming, the rest of the day was rather empty. I knew there was a swimming pool at a hotel in Great Barrington, Massachusetts. It wasn't far from Copake, probably about twenty minutes driving time. It was open to the public, and they charged only two dollars a day. Swimming put more stress on my body than I thought possible. A sauna in the same room alleviated that condition. My body had time to rest, slow down, and recoup. I enjoyed the sauna heat for as long as I could tolerate it. Afterward, the water felt exceptionally cold, an additional benefit. As good as the sauna felt, if I didn't have access to a cold swim, then there was no sauna.

The *high* I obtained from the first swim was terrific, and it was difficult to leave the pool. I felt protected from the world when I was immersed in the water. The environmental, temperature changes I struggled with daily were eliminated. I escaped the wind too. The water was a stable temperature. I didn't have to adapt to the indoor heat and the outdoor cold or the other way around.

I was able to accept the extreme difference in temperatures when going from the hot sauna to the cold pool; however, I tried to escape going from warm temperatures in a building to cold temperatures outdoors and vice versa.

This alleviated temperature changes. I didn't have to wear a lot of clothing or endure different fabrics that felt awful next to my skin. While I swam, I didn't think about food or hiding away from people as I ate. The whole experience was quiet, and it calmed my inner core to a peaceful state. When I entered the water, I was in my own kingdom, and the water was an imaginary shield that kept all discomfort at a distance.

It was as if I were a mermaid returning to the ocean after being held captive on land too long. It was here that I functioned perfectly.

Peace isn't something that exists all the time;
the important thing is to recognize it and embrace it. And I did just that.

Not only did I get a high from the cold water, but something else felt wonderfully good. As I walked into the pool, it felt as if the cold water slithered inside my sensitive areas. The feeling of intense cold against the normal heat of that part of my body was incredibly sensual. It made me feel like a woman, and I wanted more. I didn't even realize what was happening at first, but the cold caused an orgasm, my first.

In time, I realized that was what happened. I knew it was something to hide, because when they occurred, I pressed my body against the pool wall and squeezed my legs together in sheer ecstasy. I was a virgin and never dated much. This was a new experience. It never happened with warm water, only cold water.

After awhile, I drove to the pool for a total of four times a day. Swimming was the answer to my suffering. I was able to rid myself of the heat for a while. I was in love with swimming in cold water. I was hooked, and I was addicted. And, of course, the orgasms made it even more pleasurable. I looked forward to them each day.

As soon as I entered the pool area, the first thing I did was take a long, *hot* sauna. Upon leaving the sauna, I immediately entered the *cool* water. That first swim after the sauna was the only time I reached a climax. They were even more enjoyable when no one was around. It was just I in my own private pool with a sexual fantasy. I wanted them to last forever. When the water wasn't cold enough, they didn't occur, and I was disappointed. I was overtaken with this new discovery.

There was an inner force that pulled me to the pool like a magnet. I couldn't stay away; therefore, I was either on the road or in the pool for most of the day. A nice long, cold shower topped off each swim, another added compulsion. I felt I couldn't live without swimming in cold water. I had to have it. I craved it, and I couldn't eat without it. Unfortunately, the water wasn't always cold, and I was a royal pain. I made a nuisance of myself, asking and pleading for colder water. As long as the water was cold, my appetite was good.

I looked for colder and colder temperatures and warmer and warmer saunas. People often stood around and watched me swim. I was told I got up to one hundred laps during some visits to the pool.

The pool closed at half past ten. After my last swim of the day, I sat in the reception area to rest before the drive home. I could see the cocktail lounge from where I sat. On weekends, the inn featured a small band, and the first time I heard them, I thought they were Chicago. The bartender wasn't too hard on the eyes either, and I was very much attracted to him. I also met a gal my age; so after my swim, we met in the lounge six nights out of the week. My new acquaintance became a solid friendship. I eagerly looked forward to our time together, so much so that I depended upon it as much as the swimming. My new life was certainly more exciting than the one I had been living.

In the summer, I went swimming at Copake Lake during the day. Every evening, I disappeared and enjoyed my swim at the pool. After awhile, all the swimming and the nightlife was exhausting. One night, on my way home at one o'clock in the morning, I fell asleep at the wheel and drove off the side of the road, hitting the guardrail. I didn't get hurt, but the car did.

When I realized what happened, I didn't move; I felt numb. I was fortunate that a friend drove by the scene right after I hit the rail. He informed me of how dangerous my accident could have been. He told me it was a close call, and even that didn't really sink in until much later. Immediately after the accident, the only thing that entered my mind was, "I can't get to the pool. I don't have a car. What am I going to do? How do I get another car? What do I do on rainy days and cool, damp days?"

I didn't even check to see if I was hurt. Fear and panic prevailed. I was afraid I couldn't get to the pool. I thought maybe my mother would lend me her car. I had to swim at the pool to eat, not the lake; it had to be the pool. I was obsessed with that thought. Nothing else mattered. There had to be a way. All these jumbled thoughts were bouncing around in my head.

The fear of being too warm was stronger than the fear of dying.

To add fuel to the fire, I had created a situation where I overheated my body before a cold swim. At the pool, I had the sauna, and at the lake, I had the sun. On cloudy or cool days, I made the cabin very warm by stoking up the Franklin stove before jumping into the lake. I adjusted my body and behavior to cater to this obsession. I was not going to let it go.

Occasionally, I tried to eat without the cold water first. It was a total disaster that set the stage for, what felt like, an inferno burning inside my body. That was difficult to put out once it began. It never occurred to me that I might be lowering my body temperature, thus causing this *on-fire* feeling. When one's body temperature is low, it makes a person feel feverish. I didn't know this at the time.

After the accident, my car was totally out of commission. I borrowed my mother's car occasionally for short distances, and that didn't include the swimming pool. I had to make do with the lake and the stove, which escalated the stress I felt. Swimming at the pool gave me a new outlook, and now it was gone.

Time passed, and fall arrived. I left the lake and stayed with my parents in the village. I was used to living alone. I asked Dad if I could live in the apartment over his funeral home, which was next door. He agreed, to his eventual dismay. I took cold showers and ran the water for long periods of time each day. The water splattered onto the floor, and one day, it leaked into the funeral parlor downstairs. That was not a good thing.

My parents had an outdoor, heated pool. When the water temperature was cold, it was magnificent; but in the early fall, the outdoor air was rather chilly, and they turned the thermostat up. As soon as my toe hit the warm water, I felt sick, and then mad. I needed cold. I couldn't survive without cold. I begged them to turn it down, but Dad wouldn't hear of it. It was more important that my mother had a warm, relaxing swim throughout the day. (Now, I totally understand his decision.) To compensate for the pool water being too warm, I turned on the oven in the apartment. I opened the oven door to let the heat escape into the room. I made an attempt to create the heat of a summer day. This made the pool feel cooler. Then I finished with a cold shower. I had no time to waste. I ate quickly before my body had a chance to heat up once again.

During one of my daily rituals, I left the oven door open and the gas on; the oven caught on fire from grease accumulation. My father called the fire department, and they quickly arrived to put out the smoky fire. I was a mess. I was shaking all over and scared of what the outcome would be. I almost knew what the decision would be. The apartment reeked of smoke, and I had to move back in with my parents. My emotional, roller-coaster ride ended in fear. I felt guilty for the way I lived. I was afraid to let my parents see what my life was like, and I was sure I would have to vacate the apartment permanently. I felt as if I was under a physical weight from the stress.

"I allowed a fire to start in our family's building. How unthinkable. How could I have been so careless and stupid?" I asked myself.

The answer was quite obvious. I was addicted to cold water and the everlasting search to find it. I was oblivious to everything else around me. I never saw any danger. My strong desire to live sometimes created an unusual course of action, but I believed I had to push the limits in order to survive. If I had been more cautious, I could have prevented the fire. It seemed to me that I would have shriveled up and died if I hadn't followed my urges.

My parents' pool was too small for my needs. I was accustomed to the wide-open spaces of Copake Lake or an Olympic-sized pool. When I went into the water, I did some serious swimming. The small pool with its warm temperatures weren't conducive to that.

As soon as my mother's car was available, I went swimming in the Ore Pit. This was within the state park in the next town. The water was crystal clear and ice cold all summer long. I felt alive when I swam there. The only problem was staying cold until I reached home. By the time I drove back to

Copake, I was warmer than before I left. The appetite I had at the Ore Pit diminished by the time I returned home. This was depressing and unexplainable. Plus, my brain played continuous mind games. I felt stuck and frustrated with my life. I couldn't get what I needed, and I was frightened. I wanted to escape this agony. I was sure everything would be perfect, if only I could get out of Copake and go back to the pool in Great Barrington.

Before long, the warm days were far and few between. The tepid water in my parents' pool was depressing; therefore, I stopped swimming. If I stayed in the house, I felt as if I were suffocating. I walked around our one block, which was smack in the center of Copake. This didn't take the place of swimming, not by a long shot, but I was in motion. I walked every day in all kinds of weather. This, too, became an obsession. I felt cool as I walked but warm when I stopped. To compensate for the heat within my body, since I didn't have the cold water, I wore very lightweight, summer clothing. My mother made me this wonderful polyester, polka-dotted sundress that fit perfectly. I completed the outfit with my favorite skimpy sandals. The only problem was, I insisted on wearing the outfit at all times, whether it was a hot day or a cold day. I firmly established, and without any likelihood of change, that wearing this outfit produced a perfect day. The type of material certainly made the difference; I was sure of it. For years, I would only wear polyester next to my skin. In reality, cotton is much cooler, but no one could convince me of that.

One day, I became bored with the same scenery and decided to walk up Route 22. I headed north to a familiar restaurant that had opened when I was around eight or nine. On this early fall day, the weather was a little cool, but I was sure I'd be home before sundown. It was about three miles to my destination, and once there, I was eager to find someone to talk to. The owner's wife was there and tried to fix me something to eat, but all I wanted was a diet soda and conversation. I hated to leave, but the sky was now dark; and when we looked outside, there was a snow squall. Several customers offered me a ride, but I was determined to walk. I started down the road, and a few minutes later, the owner's wife was right beside me in her car. She was worried about me not having enough clothes on and walking in the very cold temperatures. She insisted on taking me home. Sometimes my brain was numb when it came to making the appropriate decisions.

Cold water swimming once a day and eventually four times a day

My father bought me another car in 1973, and I was on the road again. The winter season was well under way, and bad, road conditions could make driving hazardous; therefore, I thought it wise to find a pool as close to the house as possible.

Jug End Barn, a very well known resort at one time, was located in South Egremont, Massachusetts, about twenty minutes from our home. They had an Olympic pool and sauna that was detached from the main building. It was open to the air in the summer and covered with a huge, canvas bubble in the winter.

I went there, at least, once a day, and I swam until I couldn't take another stroke. Then I relaxed in the lounge before driving home. I was too comfortable after my evening swim, and the warmth in the room almost put me to sleep more than once.

The distance between our home and the resort became longer as the days moved along. And my parents hinted around about a job prospect at the resort. A small part of me felt guilty because I wasn't working, and the larger part wanted a job at the resort so that I was closer to the pool at all times. I had a difficult time pulling myself away from the resort each evening. I was totally at peace and content as I sat in the resort lounge. I didn't want to let go of that fulfillment. As I drove out of the parking lot and headed home, all the gratification slipped away.

At home, I wasn't able to sit and relax. My brain was never without turmoil. I attempted to be in control of the thermostat and turned down the furnace whenever I got the chance. When my father realized why the house was cooling down, he was rather stern with me. His tone frightened me at first. However, it wasn't long before I cautiously stood at the thermostat and, ever so gently, moved it just the slightest bit.

My obsessive-compulsive need to be surrounded in cold water took me farther and farther away from my family. Swimming represented a freedom I didn't have in the real world. Once I was engulfed in the water, a whole new world opened up. All my cares, worries, and fears disappeared. I swam until I was exhausted. Then all unpleasant thoughts were gone. When I returned home from the pool, I frequently had to answer to my whereabouts and why I stayed away so much.

The person I am today, I don't dispute their parental worry at all. I completely understand. But back then, the more questions there were, the more I stayed away. The more I stayed away, the less I had in common with my family. The childhood structuring appeared to be lost. I got some relief from swimming in cold water. That is all that mattered at that time in my life. I needed relief. I was sure a therapist couldn't take my *hot* feeling away. In my mind, the perfect solution for my predicament was swimming.

In order to be close to my obsession, I inquired about obtaining a job and was hired as a pastry chef assistant and a fill-in waitress. Along with the job, came room and board and full use of the pool. The whole package sounded like the ideal solution, in theory.

I moved into the resort. It was a relief to be close to the pool and have access to it any time of the day; however, each morning was a whole new story. I was still hot as I began each day, and the urgency to be in the cool water intensified. Plus, I was never absolutely sure the pool would be waiting for me. The ever-present worry and mind games: what if the pool is closed today for sanitary reasons, or someone forgot to unlock the door? Every morning began in fear, and the uncertainty caused much anxiety. I didn't have a say in what happened with the pool. It might even get shut down. Then I'd have to relocate and start a whole new routine. I was never sure of tomorrow and where I was going to swim.

The reason for swimming was to cool down. Then I could eat. My car needed to be easily accessible after the swim, because that is where I ate my meals. The distance between the pool and my room was over one hundred feet, so it was imperative I parked my car in a handy spot. Right after my swim, I made a quick exit and went straight to my vehicle. I knew the night before what I would eat for breakfast. It couldn't be perishable, because I kept it in my room on the windowsill. Then I prayed for cloudy days, so the food wouldn't spoil. Half awake and blurry-eyed in the morning, I put my items in my canvas bag, dropped them off in my car, and staggered to the pool. I could have sworn I was engulfed in a thick cloud that separated me from other people. I felt as though I were in another world that was out of focus. The division between the two didn't allow me to be part of their society.

When I immersed into the cool water, the encasement disappeared, and I joined the rest of the world. Then I was awake. The moment I finished my swim, I made a mad dash to my vehicle and prayed no one stopped me to talk. Conversation slowed me down, and that heated me up. I was sort of a Dr. Jekyll and Mr. Hyde. When I was away from the water, I was one person: very sociable and looking for company and people to talk to. When I swam, I was all business and very serious. There wasn't time for much chitchat.

The lunch I packed usually consisted of ham and cheese sandwiches, apples, yogurt, and juice. I drove to the nearest restaurant to buy hot coffee and something sweet, which was usually ice cream. Nutrition wasn't on my mind — just what tasted good, what was satisfying, and what gave me the energy to swim.

I also started smoking cigarettes. I think taking time to smoke a cigarette slowed me down for a moment. Smoking also boosted my appetite. The habit would soon prove to be dangerous. I often had a cigarette still burning as I finished up my meal, and I balanced it on the dashboard. I can't explain why, except that the swimming must have anesthetized my brain.

I guess I became so engrossed with what I ate; it was as if I were in a trance. I never ate one morsel of food without swimming first. The whole process took many steps before I could sit down and begin a meal. Once I was in the process of eating, I tried to take in as much food as possible. As a result, I just didn't pay attention to the burning cigarette. After awhile, I had burn marks all over the dashboard. There wasn't any way to hide them. I embarrassed myself with such actions. Thank goodness, no one else ever saw my car. This is *not* how I was raised.

Most of the pool people were friendly. Several seemed to want more then a brief encounter, but I didn't let anyone get too close. An exchange of a few words in the sauna, with whoever happened to be sitting there, was about the extent of any conversation. I didn't make any plans. My life was a day-to-day existence and one I did not understand. I certainly didn't expect anyone else to comprehend this bizarre behavior. The reality of it all was overwhelming. Each day was a never-ending routine I wasn't able to stop.

Occasionally, after finishing a meal in my car, I sat there clenching the steering wheel with both hands. Tears rolled down my cheeks as I thought, "Why me? What has happened? How did I get here? How can I fix this? I am falling into a deep hole, a very negative dark and gloomy hole."

Then I'd snap out of the mood, even though I continued to do the same thing over and over. I was not going to be defeated. This would not destroy me. I would make it through this mess somehow.

Recently, while watching the movie *Things We Lost in the Fire*, I heard an addict say something that hit home. It seemed to connect with this period of my life. It went something like this: The first high is the best, the ultimate fulfillment of what one is expecting and more; after that, it is never the same, and you're always looking for it.

I believe this reference was to drugs and getting high. My addiction to cold water was very similar. The beginning was amazing. When it became a need, not a pleasure, the enjoyment lessened. As it took over my life, it became a disaster.

When I had a few days off, I drove to Cape Cod and visited my sister. Staying with other people was a challenge. I tried to hide my split personality. Upon my arrival, I was happy and talkative and tried to act like nothing was wrong with me.

As soon as I opened my eyes in the morning, I was a furnace. I had to get to cold water as fast as possible. I always awakened before anyone else. I dressed, grabbed my gear, left quietly, and went searching for a pool. Not being from the area, plus coping with traffic while the sun's rays burned against my skin, plus trying to find a hotel with a pool, reality set in.

I thought, "What if there isn't a pool? I'll never make it, driving all over the area just to find a pool. What if they stop me from going swimming? I hope no one talks to me. Please, let the water be ice cold. Will there be a place to take a shower? When I'm done, will my car be near the building? I hope I can eat before anyone sees me. I should have never come."

I was lucky and found a hotel with a pool. I parked the car. The next challenge was being allowed to swim. I didn't seek permission; I used the pool as if I were a guest. I didn't carry out this act as a prank. I summed it up as a necessity, and that was that.

I was afraid to just *take off* and do something out of my element, especially without a concrete plan. Occasionally, I just did it, but it wasn't without stress. The anticipation of the trip was exciting, because it was away from my obsessive-compulsive behavior. Yet, I brought my actions along, and spontaneity was close to nonexistent in my life.

I stayed at the cape, and away from my job, a little too long. Upon returning to the resort, I was fired.

Chapter 6
Del's House

Jug End Barn wasn't too far from the inn where I used to swim. Immediately, after I was fired, I drove into Great Barrington. My first priority was to find a pool. I went straight to my old, stomping ground: the inn. The new, desk clerk was my friend from the past. It was great to see her.

The good ol' days drifted back into my thoughts. It was after my last swim of the day that I came alive. I was free to socialize. My friend and I met in the cocktail lounge and spent an hour or so listening to the rock band. Both of us were unemployed and the night was ours. I took a reasonable interest in my evening clothes. A casual, but form fitting, mid-length, denim skirt was accompanied by a white, long-sleeved, polyester blouse revealing enough creamy white skin on the neckline, and finished off with a sporty, navy vest.

I dressed to catch someone's eye. If I was lucky, I'd be asked to dance. If not, it didn't take much to encourage either one of us to dance. The beat of the music took over my body as if I were born dancing. Even though I wasn't a good dancer, it didn't matter. A song began to play and, instantaneously, my foot tapped the floor, next, a little movement in the hips to the right, and then the left. With eyes closed, I hummed the melody, and then out came the words. I was sure feelin' the music and couldn't wait to be out on the floor and let everything go. When I was in high school two females were often seen dancing together. If at all possible, we didn't want to sit when we heard the music. As I grew older I was a little more hesitant. However, during this stage of my life, I was less concerned about what people thought or said. There was no way I would sit out a dance and lose that moment of elation. I only ordered ice water. I wasn't there to drink, plus the mornings were difficult enough. I didn't need alcohol. My friend had her eye on a band member; I was attracted to the bartender.

On my return, the energy between us was different. It was now 1974, and my friend had her life in order; I didn't. She had a job, an apartment, and was fashionably dressed in business clothes. She was very kind but distant. I explained my dilemma. She said there was a room where a couple had just checked out. Room service wouldn't be in there until tomorrow, and I could spend one night. It was extremely generous of her. She could have lost her job.

I was close to the pool. It was a blissful ending to a stressful day. Before each meal, I went for a swim. Then one more dip after dinner. I was at the lounge as soon as it opened, eager to hear some great music and dance. The same bartender was on duty, which made it more appealing.

I didn't tell her, and she trusted me enough not to check, but I remained in the room past that one night. One afternoon, I had the shock of my life. The pool was shut down and posted as unsanitary. The pool in front of me was filled with water. I was addicted to swimming. I was not concerned about the condition. I had to swim. I waited until after dark, then checked out several windows until I found one I could open. The water was still, discolored, and stagnant.

The room was dark and even smelled musty. I kept a close eye on the front desk in order to plan my entry and not be seen. My friend wasn't working that night. I entered the pool room, quickly slipped into the water, and eagerly began to swim. It wasn't a long swim that night. I was way too nervous. I grabbed my towel and climbed out the window and scurried to my room. Soon after, my friend realized I had not vacated the room, and she questioned me. I told her the truth; I had stayed for a week. I wasn't charged for the room but was promptly asked to leave.

I should have realized this was a wakeup call for me. Not only was my behavior affecting my life but also threatened the livelihood of my friend. She was hurt by what I did, but being loyal, she told me I could spend one night on her sofa. The next evening, we went to another lounge in town, where a friend of hers played the piano.

I was introduced to a beautiful, female singer named Del Rae. I adored Del the moment we met. She had a soft and gentle way about her, was friendly, and easy to talk to. I was in awe of her talent and poise. We talked, and she told me she had an extra room if I wanted to stay at her home. I quickly accepted and moved in. I spent a good deal of the day at the pool, but when we were together, we had some wonderful moments. It wasn't long before she called me her little sister. Del was easy to love. She tried to understand what was happening to me and wanted to help. I was on my own in this predicament, yet it was nice knowing she was there for me when I needed company and someone to talk with.

Del and her husband always included me in their activities. Neither one of us had any money. She had left New York City to get away from the fast pace and enjoy some leisure time in the Berkshires. She had a small gig at a restaurant in town; however, money was limited. My job consisted of swimming every day, and that didn't bring in any income.

The Christmas holiday was approaching, and we were broke, but we were happy with the bond that developed between us. It was important to me because my behavior caused me to distance myself from my own family. One afternoon, we talked about Christmas trees. I reminisced about the family tradition of searching for the perfect long needle, pine tree. We took Del's car and found our way to the property of one of my relatives who owned a farm very close to Del's house. We found the most beautiful tree in the forest. Del actually cut the tree down herself, and I was doubly impressed. We decorated it with the few ornaments she had in storage, and it became a cherished memory. In the years that followed, this simple event was always part of the conversation.

We had each other, a roof over our heads, and laughter in the house; we didn't seem to need much more.

Her friendship didn't conquer my addiction. I still needed to swim.

My favorite inn closed their pool in 1975. This specific building and pool was an important part of my existence. I didn't want to let it go. I agonized over the news and complained excessively to anyone who would listen. Of course, that didn't get me anywhere.

Nearby was another resort, and they had two pools: a small, indoor and a large, outdoor pool. This was the only spot I could find. I was impatient when I stood at the front desk waiting for someone to take the two-dollar, swimming fee. The lobby was hot, and my stomach was queasy. I knew once I was in the pool, I would find some relief; and, for a brief time, all would be right with the world. I was devastated as soon as my toe touched the water. The water was bathtub warm. I felt as if my heart sank to the bottom of the pool. Thoughts dashed through my mind.

"This is my third pool, and this one stinks. Where else can I go? I have no choice. I'll just have to put up with it and figure out a way to make it feel cooler. Darn it, swimming at the inn was so good. Why did it end? I'm a wreck. How can other people swim in this and like it?"

The sauna helped make the water feel a little cooler, but not much. I always ended the swim with an extremely long, cold shower. So long, people waiting got very annoyed. Then I quickly dressed, dashed out to my car, and ate. In very warm weather, I returned to the dressing room to take another cold shower. When exiting, there were these huge grates in the side of one wall where strong, moving air poured out. When I finished my shower, I stood in front of them with eyes closed. I hung on to every wave of cool air, as if it were my last, before finally leaving the building. I frequented here four times a day, starting with the first swim at six thirty in the morning and the last at nine o'clock in the evening.

This pool was very small and not nearly as cold as I needed. The daily attempt to make myself cold wasn't successful. The cooling process became more difficult and complicated.

My constant complaints about the warm water were a waste of time; they didn't care at all. I was ignored and barely tolerated. I think they could have done very nicely without my two-dollar-a-day business. I spent endless time in the shower, using as much of the resort's cold water as possible. I stayed in the sauna longer and longer. I was to control the pool water temperature.

One time, the owner found me asleep in the sauna. He shouted at me with anger tone in his voice, "I want the timer set." With a very serious look on his face, he informed me that I terrified him and then proceeded to lecture me on the danger of staying in a sauna too long.

I knew the lifestyle I lived wasn't normal, and I certainly wasn't proud of it. I knew everyone around me recognized my behavior as unusual, at best. The addiction had me, and I didn't know how to break away.

One of the local churches offered a free service to those in need of therapy for whatever reason. An acquaintance suggested I make an appointment. He thought it might help me; I wasn't so sure. I went a few times. I talked briefly about the obsession to swim in cold water and why. Even while I sat there with him, the *why* was obvious, at least, to me. I was overcome with a feeling of tremendous heat; nothing changed. The only thing I wanted to do was flee his office and be in the cool, fresh air. I tried to please someone else by seeking therapy, but it didn't please me. It seemed senseless to continue with the sessions.

Unfortunately, the addiction to cold water took me away from society. When I was ready to socialize, others retired for the day or went to work. A schedule for most people is generally wrapped around their job or home life. I had neither. What I did have was an obsession, which had it's own agenda. I allowed it to dictate the free time.

The real *me* loved being around people, on my timetable. When people were kind and made me laugh, I clung to the hope of a lasting friendship. I was heartbroken when I had to detach myself from anyone, for whatever the reason.

Then there was that other woman in my head. She tried to hide the addiction and make people believe she was fine. She wasn't fine. She was very unhappy on some days and projected a lot of negative, internal dialogue. The addiction was always present.

Swimming was exciting and fulfilling in the beginning. When it became a compulsion and a driving force, it was not pleasurable anymore. I dreaded the swimming routine. The choice of going or not going was no longer a factor in the equation; I was addicted. I sank deeper into a black hole and saw no way out.

My friend, Del, was waiting for a record to be recorded at a small studio nearby. When the time came, she needed my room for some of the musicians. We talked, and she felt bad about asking me to leave, but it had to be. Music was her career.

She previously resided in an old hotel in Great Barrington. I decided my best move was to check the place out. The drive to the pool and back to the hotel would take over twenty minutes each way, but my options were few.

Chapter 7
Room with No View

The hotel certainly wasn't the Ritz. It had a bar and cocktail lounge for weekend music but no restaurant. The entire upstairs was rented out to low-income people. My single room wasn't much: a small, bleak room with a bathroom. There was a twin bed in one corner. I added a card table and one chair. I prepared the table as if someone were going to eat. I pretended that someday a meal would be enjoyed here — a wishful thought. I actually sat at the table a few times; however, I didn't eat one morsel of food in my apartment. I wanted to create a homey atmosphere so when all my swimming was done for the day, I had something to come home to; but nothing I created helped.

The building was infested with cockroaches. Every evening, when I turned on the bathroom light, I saw them scatter and run for the drain. It was a good thing I did all my bathing at the pool. There was no way I would get into the bathtub where bugs lurked. Every month, the tenants received a notice about fumigating the entire building on a such and such a date. I imagined how unhealthy that was, the thought of the chemical being used around the entire room; it gave me the creeps. I guess it was the only way to keep the *critters* under control, but the smell was awful, and I didn't even want to sleep there.

When a fuse blew, maintenance replaced it with a penny to complete the power grid. I remembered my father saying it wasn't a good idea to fix the outage with a coin. When I mentioned it to the custodian, I was told that was how they did things there.

Staying cool was my main concern, as was having my small, air conditioner work. For the most part, the penny only lasted a short time before another fuse blew. The fear of not knowing how long a fuse would last kept me in a state of panic during the hot weather. I pleaded, like an insane woman, to the custodian. Fear and need placed me in a vulnerable position. I was desperate. He was popular with many women, and he could have easily taken advantage of me. Thank God, he didn't.

Wherever I landed, day or night, those thoughts never crossed my mind. My brain didn't seem to have the capacity for danger. I could have been raped or beat up or, worse yet, killed. Many nights, I was out until 4 a.m. I often visited friends who kept late hours or worked the late shift. I was desperate to talk to anyone once my ritual was over. I had a one-track mind:

staying cold and doing what I thought I had to do. Nothing else mattered.

There were people coming and going at all hours of the night at the hotel. Each neighbor could hear just about everything that went on, which wasn't always pleasant.

I never lived in such conditions, but it didn't seem to bother me a whole lot. The people were friendly, and that was more important. Most of the day, I was out of the room while I swam and ate my meals. When I returned, it was depressing. I missed Del, and I was lonely.

When I wasn't swimming, I walked up and down the sidewalk aimlessly. I loved to walk, but people looked at me as if I were weird. On rainy days, I walked inside. One time, I was in a shop, and the owner approached me. She said if I wasn't going to buy anything to, please, leave. I'm sure now, she thought I was shoplifting. That thought was never on my mind then. Walking made me feel happier and cooler.

I could have functioned very nicely without the sun. It only made my life more difficult. I was already too warm. The heat of the sauna was fine, but not the sunshine. Cloudy, moderately warm days were the best when indoors matched the outdoors.

I often visited a pharmacy/coffee shop with no intention of eating but just went for the company. I teamed up with the most unusual group of individuals. They turned out to be really good friends. Some of them were shunned by society for their appearance. They frequented this store just to have egg malts and talk. I joined them for what seemed to be hours, talking and laughing. They were all heart and soul, and enjoyable to be around. They didn't care that I swam most of the day or if I wore the same outfit each time they saw me. They didn't judge me. I knew I could always count on them if I needed a place to hang my hat, a place to get out of the weather for a few hours, or just needed someone to talk to. They listened and cared. My visits were always brief. I never stayed in one spot too long. As soon as my body started to feel warm, I took off for the pool.

I wore the same clothes day in and day out. Style wasn't important. I didn't have them on very long before I changed into my swimsuit. When I wore a specific outfit and had a good day, I continued to wear the same outfit for days, then months, and then years. Fashion and variety didn't matter — only comfort.

All the stress I developed in school over clothing choices was gone now. I eliminated decisions. I just wore the same items.

Heavy clothing attributed to the heat I felt. My summer outfit was a sundress and sandals. I wore the ensemble from March to the end of October. I didn't look forward to wearing winter clothing; and even then, my attire consisted of a lightweight skirt, polyester top, and a raincoat. On the coolest days of the year, I added another lightweight garment for layers, which could easily be removed. I always dreaded adding more clothes, especially a hat and boots. I got caught one time in a snowstorm with sandals. I was finally convinced summer was over.

The odd thing was, I didn't realize something like this would be an issue with other people. Why the stares? Why the whispers? Why the avoidance? One time, while I was in the swimming pool, a group of teenage girls threw my clothes into a large, waste can. I went to the locker room and couldn't find my clothes anywhere. When I did find them, the girls giggled and ran out the door. When times are tough, why is it some people want to spoil another person's day and make them feel worse?

I was in my own world, with a very rigid daily plan. There was no question in my mind that the day would not begin unless I was able to swim. I lost credibility, and respect. My whole lifestyle and existence was so unorthodox, even the few friends I had — other than the coffee shop gang — didn't trust me, as I was soon to find out.

When I moved into town, I was introduced to a friendly couple. Many visits followed, and I found them quite enjoyable. I was asked to house sit for two days while they went away, and I agreed; but when the couple returned, I was accused of stealing money. It was a very awkward situation and an unfair assessment. They knew me well enough to believe me. I felt it was convenient for them to put the blame on me. I was an easy target because I was unemployed and had rather unusual habits, by their standards. I thought these people were my friends. I was infinitely wronged and deeply hurt.

I purchased most of my groceries before each meal. Breakfast had to be handy when I left for the pool, so I kept what I could on the windowsill just as I had in the past.

Daybreak was extremely difficult, close to a nightmare. As the morning light shone across my apartment floor, I struggled to open each eye. My eyelids were heavy, and the bright light made me squint. Once awake, I had to get out of bed because I felt as though someone had turned on the heat. This was a natural sensation every morning, even if the room was cool. The warmth I felt rushed up my spine and engulfed my head. Instantly, I pushed my imaginary *panic button*.

The routine never changed much. I got dressed, grabbed my food, locked the door behind me, and made my way to the car. The process wasn't any better, and now I lived in a place where I was more likely to bump into people. Acquaintances saw the real me at night: alert, smiling, talkative, and bouncing about. I was embarrassed to have them catch a glimpse of my sad state of affairs. As I left the premises, I was definitely in a state of disorientation and struggled to walk.

All the days ran together into a blur of indescribable confusion and chaos. I had no control over my life. My body just went through the motions. I put food in my mouth to stay alive, and very little at that. The whole scenario was a nightmare just waiting for the ball to drop. And I was gaining weight again. One of my friends suggested I see a doctor. I didn't have any money, but I made an appointment. I don't remember how or if I paid him. The doctor wouldn't give me diet pills but prescribed Valium. He thought it would help the anxiety and the panic I experienced in the morning hours. I hesitated but decided to give them a try. I thought a pill might help numb my brain.

I took one before leaving the apartment each morning. The pill slowed me down, but it didn't take away the heat. I continued with the same obsessive behavior; only now I had the after effects of the pill to deal with. Moving one foot in front of the other was difficult. It was as if I had extra weight on each foot and a strong force pulling me to a sitting position. I clutched the stair rails and almost stumbled down each step. I groped my way until I reached the exit and then made my way to my car. There I sat for a few minutes and waited for the fuzziness in my head to depart. When I thought it was safe, I drove to the pool.

The panic attacks lessened, but navigating was another story. Once I started ingesting the pills, I couldn't give them up. The doctor refilled them only once. I was addicted to those now, too. I kept asking for more, but he refused. I pleaded and begged. The receptionist said she'd have to call the police if I didn't stop coming.

In my mind, I knew I had to go through every part of the cold-water addiction over and over again. I couldn't get off this merry-go-round. It wasn't merry at all. It was exhausting. I was drowning in this huge, slippery bowl of cold water. Yet, the cold water was the only thing that gave me a life.

By the time I arrived at the pool, the medication was working. It gave me a comfortable, cozy feeling. I didn't want to move out of the car. The struggle and conflict between *my* and *self* — I viewed *myself* as two people: my, *the real me* and self, *the addicted me* — continued, although it was muted by the medication. The real me wanted to stop and live like a normal, human being. The addicted one could not eat without swimming and taking several cold showers. Every day, I made my body go through this torturous, obsessive behavior.

Occasionally, when I wasn't swimming, I went for a drive into Copake and made an attempt to spend some time with my parents. I was uncomfortable and ashamed to stay very long. This new lifestyle wasn't anything to be proud of. It certainly was not the way I was brought up. My everyday attire was acceptable to me, but I knew it didn't sit well with my parents the first time I visited. About halfway to Copake, I pulled over on the side of the road and slipped into something more appropriate. I knew it would make my mother happy if she saw me wearing the corduroy, wrap-around skirt she made me. I added a conservative, crisp, white blouse to match. I didn't like wearing either one. As soon as the skirt touched my body, I began to heat up. It was as if the skirt contained heat all the time and was waiting to release it into a body. I looked at these kinds of clothes as the enemy. I didn't want any part of them. All I wanted to do was get into my comfy, cool clothes so I could be me. In this outfit, I was somebody they wanted me to be. I avoided going to visit as much as possible; I dreaded becoming too warm. I knew them well enough to know I put a lot of stress and worry on them. I know it was heartless behavior, yet my brain seemed oblivious to the pain I caused. Instead, I was zoned in on my own pain and survival. When I wasn't ill, I felt guilty about putting them through such a difficult time.

Throughout this period, my parents paid for almost all expenses, especially my room and gas, which I was totally grateful for. I can't imagine what my life would have been without this money. I should probably have been on assistance, but I didn't know anything about it.

After one of these rare jaunts, I was on the way back to my rented room when I decided to stop at a familiar restaurant. I thought I recognized a car, and I was in the mood to see a friendly face of someone I once knew. I found an old friend sitting at the snack bar. I didn't order anything, but we had a good time talking and laughing. But on the way out, I fell on the gravel parking lot.

My knee was loaded with small stones and moderately painful. Once again, the fear of not being able to swim took preference on the worry list, and I was inclined to ignore the injury. I didn't want to be alone, so I went to a friend's apartment. She suggested I go to the emergency room, and in fact, she insisted on driving me there.

I hesitated, but I knew it needed attention, so I went with her. An ER attendant removed all of the stones and then cleaned the wound. My heart sank when I was told I needed stitches, and then the doctor gave me specific directions; both didn't fit into my lifestyle. It was imperative I keep the wound clean and dry for a couple of days. I wanted to turn back the clock. I could have done quite nicely without falling in the first place, and this wasn't going to help my daily routine at all. By the time my friend and I left the ER, it was very late in the day. I missed my evening swim, which, by choice, led to no dinner.

I was a total mess and incredibly stressed. The way I acted, it's a wonder we both didn't have a heart attack. She asked me to stay with her until I calmed down, and it was close to bedtime. That way, I had something to do that would pass the time and, hopefully, take my mind off missing my last swim of the day.

Once I was back at my own place, I watched the clock most of the night, waiting for the morning to arrive.

I drove to the pool and tried to slither past the management. Quietly, and without being noticed, I edged down into the water. I got in one lap before the owner of the resort saw the bandage.

He said, "No swimming with that bandage on you. There will be no open wounds in this pool, and I don't want to see you swimming until it is healed."

I was so scared, the blood rushed to my head, and I stood there frozen.

"Now what?" I thought. "There has to be a way to swim. I could try once more. That wouldn't be wise; the owner was as sharp as a tack."

I was desperate. I found a brook on the property, some distance from the main building. There was barely enough water to cover me in a horizontal position, but at least, it was ice cold. It was foolish and in direct conflict with my doctor's orders, but my addiction drove me to a total lack of concern for such trivial matters. I don't think the owner really wanted me up there; nevertheless, he didn't stop me.

When the wound healed, I returned to the indoor pool but found it way too hot. Day after day, I swam in the outdoor pool. It, too, was very warm, not refreshing, and did nothing to cool me down. I swam in it anyway. Each day, when I arrived, I prayed for cold water. I watched all the other customers smiling and having such a good time. They were there to relax and float around in the water. My needs were different. I swam as a means of survival, not for fun. I wanted to be smiling, too, but it never happened in that dreadful, warm water. When I departed each day, I was mad at the world, sour, and uncomfortably hot — not a good combination.

Chapter 8
The Bartender

My days were pretty much occupied with swimming and meals. I grumbled continuously about the temperature of the water, which only added to my stress level and put a damper on my personality. My deep-rooted thought of having to stop what I was doing, drive to a pool, swim, shower, and eat was over for the day. I looked forward to socializing with people who had a normal routine. I was ready to come alive, but most everyone else was in bed except for the night crowd.

The same bartender still worked at the inn where my friend and I went in the past. My final swim of the day was out of the way, and I could relax for the rest of the evening. It was then that I looked for conversation and a few hours of companionship. Most evenings, I frequented the lounge and sat at the bar talking with the bartender. I never drank alcohol. I was there for the music and for his presence.

There wasn't a cocktail waitress working the lounge. I offered to help serve drinks without pay. In truth, it gave me an excuse to hang around until the bartender closed up shop. Plus, I felt needed. I learned the routine quickly and made a few tips, which made the job more exciting. Each night, the bartender gave me a five-or ten-dollar bill out of his tips, and it came in handy for groceries. The atmosphere was completely different from my daily routine, and I easily forgot about swimming for a few hours. I was easily attracted to this environment where people were smiled, laughed, and had a good time.

My infatuation for the bartender was intense, and throughout the day, I thought about the moment when I'd see him again. I was drawn to him like the sun soaks up water. When I was in his presence, I felt different — like a real woman. In the past, I was afraid he might see me eating in my car or picking up on my swimming routine. I didn't want that to happen, so I always parked my car out of view. I wanted him to know the person I once was and wanted to be, not the addicted one.

Being around this guy was the best part of my day. He was *Clark Gable handsome*, for starters. In his company, I felt as if I were smiling on the inside. We spent more and more time together, and one evening, he invited me back to his apartment. We ended up lying on his bed and talking for a while. Then we fell asleep in each other's arms.

Another night after work, we went to a nearby bar. The music filled the air with a romantic gesture, and my new flame asked me to dance. He held me close; our bodies moved in unison. I closed my eyes and thought I was in heaven. I pressed my body closer to his, and he became aroused. He told me we had to sit down, and I questioned him as to why. I, at twenty-eight years old, didn't even know what just happened. When I came to my senses, I wondered how I could have been so stupid and naive.

The thought of sex turned me on, but the actual fear of it was frightening. All my adolescent insecurities were present in the mind of a full-grown woman. I had no experience in lovemaking. Even a book couldn't explain every situation. I withdrew from this part of my life. Now it was approaching like a freight train; would I be ready?

In spite of my fears and unanswered questions, I asked the bartender back to my tiny, nothing apartment. I didn't have a clue as to what was going to happen; however, I had hopes. There wasn't anything else to do in this empty mausoleum but go to bed. And the bed was very small. He was, at least, six feet four inches, and I was five feet nine inches. There wasn't much room to spare.

There was room for my addiction and need to be cold. As a result, the window in my apartment was open at all times, especially in winter when the building had the heat on. It was open that night.

We lay together on my small, twin bed. Just lying there made me feel special. The thought of someone wanting me made me feel beautiful inside and out. I was a bit nervous as the reality of it all sunk into my mind. "Do I move first?" I knew whatever I did would be wrong. I had butterflies in my stomach, and my nerves were uncontrollable. I had to believe this was going to be my time, a night I'd never forget and the best moment of my life. He brought himself over to me, and we started to make love. I was on fire, but not in the usual way. Nothing else mattered. I closed my eyes and couldn't believe it was actually me in the bed, lying next to a *drop-dead* handsome man.

Then, in the heat of the moment, he said, "It's too damn cold in here. I have to get out of this frigid room."

Have you ever been rejected because the room was too cold? He left, and I was ashamed and alone. I was angry, because my illness spoiled the moment. My special encounter didn't happen. I can justify it now and say the ending was probably a blessing in disguise. Protection wasn't even on my mind, and I didn't need to be pregnant at that time in my life.

After my disastrous night, the bartender knew more about me than I wanted to share, and we didn't see much of each other thereafter. I avoided his bar and lost the main outlet for socialization I had.

Chapter 9
Darkness Again

My behaviors were noticed. The desk clerk at the resort became less friendly and inattentive. The owner approached me and said it would be better if I found another place to swim; I was upsetting the guests. The pool was too warm anyway. There was one aggravation after another. This was one more on the list.

There was one song that played constantly on the public announcement system. The year was 1975, and it seemed to last forever. I believe Jackie DeShannon just released the song "Bette Davis Eyes." The resort must have enjoyed the melody and the words. I swam there, at least, four times a day, and each time I went, I heard "Bette Davis Eyes." Maybe it was just the association that led me to find the song annoying. I often mumbled to myself, "If I hear 'Bette Davis Eyes' one more time,..." To this day, I'm unable to listen to that song without the bad memories haunting me.

There was no time to waste. I needed to find a pool for the next day. The YWCA in Pittsfield, Massachusetts, was my only option. The drive was much longer and took thirty-five minutes one way. I had to park on the side street. It's amazing how an addiction gave me the strength to do things I might not ordinarily choose to do. I didn't like this new arrangement, yet water was water, and I had no other alternative.

Swimming in cold water was my number one priority. It was more important than meeting friends and family, dating, or socializing. Who would get involved with a woman that lived in a pool of cold water and needed cold for her brain to function?

I rarely saw my family. We grew more distant as time passed. I knew very little, next to nothing, of what happened in their lives. I was embarrassed by my behavior and didn't make any effort to communicate with them. I knew what the conversation would be, and so I rarely allowed them into my life. Each day, not knowing probably hurt them more than I'll ever know.

I was oblivious to the feelings of my family. I was so consumed with my own pain and addiction, I left no room for them. All through these rough times, my parents continued to pay for my rent and car needs. My running tab at the grocery store ended after I left my father's apartment. My parents felt the spending was way out of control for one person. When I think back, I don't know how I did it financially. Whatever little I needed to survive, God provided it from somewhere or someone. I never went hungry. Clothes and home furnishings weren't on my mind. Survival, under the terms of my addiction, was the single most important aspect of my life. People commented that more money would make my life a little easier. I disagreed. Money was not going to eliminate my need for cold water.

If I needed a bath, the pool water at the YWCA would have been perfect. It was unhealthy warm. The obsessive thoughts in my head escalated and stressed me out even more. I yearned for the days when I spent less time on the road and had invigorating, cold water to swim in at any hour of the day. The inn had been perfect. There was none of that here.

The YWCA didn't offer an evening swim, and that made my life even more problematical. I was determined to swim and shower three times a day before each meal. That meant I had to eat my meals closer together because the pool closed in the late afternoon. I no sooner finished one meal, and I was back at the pool for another meal even when I wasn't hungry. I was also used to swimming a lot of laps, but not here. The warm water made everyone look as if he or she were hypnotized and bobbing around like a buoy. I wasn't about to join this society. A pool was meant to swim in. This wasn't exercise. Each day, I felt as if my life was being taken away from me. I was unable to reason out anything in my head. I was mad at whoever was in charge of all the swimming pools I frequented. No one could give me a good reason why the pool was warm. And it created bacteria. If for no other reason, the health board should have recognized that. And because the water was extremely warm, I was dizzy and nauseous when I exited the pool. I struggled each day with the conditions, trying to make it work on my behalf.

I continued with the long, cold showers, hoping to compensate for the warm water. The cold shower was more important than ever. It had to imitate how my body felt when I swam in cold water. I closed my eyes and imagined I was in the pool. Often, I stepped out of the shower and re-entered just to get a little more cold water. I didn't want to separate myself from the water. I probably would have tried eating in the shower if I thought I could get away with it.

The days were getting colder, and I was becoming warmer. My daily attire was very light, summer clothing topped with an inadequately thin, shabby, raincoat. I was sure my head would heat up before I reached my car, so just before leaving the locker room, I soaked a towel with cold water. I wrapped it around my head and quickly made an exit to my car, which was parked on the side street. It was winter, and with the snow blowing in all directions, the wetness of each flake made my body feel even colder. Most people were hurrying to get out of the cold; I welcomed it. I turned the heat off in the car and rolled a window completely down. With the cold, dripping wet towel still on my head, I proceeded to eat a meal.

When my body was chilled to the bone and my fingers were turning white, my appetite was great. My menu didn't vary; I lived on ham and cheese sandwiches with lots of butter, occasionally an apple, hot coffee, ice cream, and cheesecake — this menu would never exist if I were eating in the warm indoors. Healthy diet, maybe not, yet I truly believe that menu is what kept me alive. And for the most part, it stabilized my body temperature until the outside temperatures really began to plummet. Sometimes, the weather was very dangerous. I had to wait in the YWCA lounge until it was safe to go back to my apartment. And there were other times, when I hung around to take up unoccupied time. My mental and physical life was exhausting, stressful, and depressing. I had little contact with my friends; there wasn't time. I was consumed with my passion. I was alone in this spiral downward hell.

I still didn't know what was wrong, or why I was forced to live like this. I gave up trying to find the answer. In my heart, I believed it was medical; something was making me so terribly hot, I couldn't endure staying indoors for any length of time. And forget eating inside a building. That possibility was out of the question. My obsessive behavior swallowed up most of the day. I wasn't in love with my day-to-day existence; it was rather grueling, but the most stressful part was the water temperature. Over and over, I repeated the same words day in and day out, "If the water in the pool was cold, then I could manage." I heard this sentence continuously and convinced myself it was all I needed in order to make it through the day.

In my opinion, my urge to swim didn't come from depression or a physiological ailment. I wanted to eat and not be hot when I ate. That was it in a nutshell. My actions may have appeared to be psychiatric. For example, I barely wore enough clothes in the winter months to keep warm. It was not an intelligent choice. The horrible warmth I felt overruled sanity.

The body loses a large amount of heat through the top of the head. I was lowering my body temperature, and it was a miracle I didn't kill myself. At the time, I didn't even think about it. Maybe I survived because a higher power was watching over me. I identified the first stages of the addiction as beginning when I was twenty years of age. I was now twenty-nine years old. My body was exhausted, and this existence was robbing me of my life.

The year was 1976 and it was one of my usual days at the YWCA. I entered the water and felt a terrible tightness around my neck when I started to swim. I continued with the breaststroke and made an attempt to submerge my entire body under the water. The pressure in my head was so intense I wasn't able to continue. Swimming just didn't feel right. I quickly exited the pool, dressed without the usual cold shower, and made my way to the lobby. I had to sit and rest. I wasn't able to push my body any further. I believed the unpleasant sensation would pass. A person beside me asked if I was okay. I answered I was fine, and then I passed out.

The desk clerk called an ambulance, and I remembered nothing until I woke up at the hospital, which, ironically, was almost in view of the YWCA. After I was a patient for a few days, a doctor took a big chunk out of my leg. He wanted to test for lupus. The test was negative. From what I remember, my vitals must have been normal. Evidently, low body temperature wasn't the case, or it wasn't low enough, or the warm hospital and nutrition elevated it. The attending doctor concluded there was nothing wrong medically. I was transferred to the psychiatric ward, and that became a nightmare.

I was totally trapped within four walls. I was hot all the time, and there was no swimming. I was a little confused, and I wasn't sure if I even wanted to see any water. I ate very little, refused drugs, or hid them. I rejected a warm shower. Cold swims and cold showers were all I knew. The mere thought of taking a warm shower — and no way to cool off — was inconceivable. It wasn't long before I had an attendant standing over me, demanding I take a shower. It was warm, obviously. All my heartfelt reasons didn't convince her; she stood by the shower compartment and made sure I went into the stall. Then the attendant watched as I turned on the water. I could have made the Guinness Book of World Records for taking the quickest shower ever.

The days in the psychiatric ward reminded me of a movie. I was playing the part of a patient with no choice, no voice, and no rights. I was down in a pit with no way out. The days were long and boring, and there was nothing to do but sit around and wait for the day to end. My parents visited me once. We had very little to say to one another. The silence was awkward, and the sentences weren't much better — empty and meaningless.

It was an unfortunate and sad existence. They couldn't find a physiological cause for the heat I felt, but I knew it was very real. I was struggling with the heat plus an unusual addiction. I was never asked to talk about what was bothering me or to prove to the doctors my condition wasn't psychiatric; there weren't any discussion groups. The staff handed out drugs, and the patients sat and drifted to who knows where.

Unfortunately, with swimming eliminated, the addiction became more complicated, because I wasn't eating much either.

My once-happy and close-knit family was now torn apart. None of us knew how to fix it. I wanted the old days back. Since that wasn't going to happen, we took one day at a time, but I was going nowhere fast. The hospital discharged me, and nothing was accomplished. In my mind, the staff did nothing but keep me from cold water. Now, it was on record that I'd been in a psychiatric ward, lovely.

My mother transported me to Copake. The ride home was quiet and tense. I knew another unpleasant adjustment was about to occur. I would be living with my family once again. I got away with eating as little as possible in the hospital. I wasn't sure if it would be that simple at home. The lifestyle I lived was extremely abnormal. How was I going to eat a meal without swimming first?

With the tremendous heat I felt, plus the lack of nutrition, I was positive I'd be back in another hospital in the future.

When the need for cold-water swimming first began, I didn't consider it an addiction. I told myself it was a survival technique. Then I saw how swimming took over my life, yet it still didn't sink in as to the severity. When I realized how truly addicted I was, I still wouldn't use the word *addicted*. I accepted it as a way of life — probably a lifestyle that would follow me to the end of time. I didn't see any danger. Rather than cure me, the hospital visit forced my addiction to adjust.

In 1976 to 1978 I began taking cold sponge baths three times a day prior to a meal. No showers and no regular full body bath in a tub of warm water.

That other voice was still in my head, saying, "Bathe your entire body in cold water, and then you can eat." That thought pattern ruled for months, which turned into years.

I left the water days behind, as far as swimming was concerned, but somehow, I had to cool my skin prior to a meal. I had to find a more acceptable substitute. Therefore, I began sponge bathing in cold water. At this point, it already looked like an addiction, and in fact, it was.

I wasn't satisfied with a quick sponge bath. Oh no, I went over my entire body with cold water three times at each session. The ritual turned into an obsessive-compulsive behavior. The cold water only kept me cool temporarily; therefore, I was always looking for more.

My hair was a component in the cooling process as well. Now long, it clung to my neck and fell toward my face. This also contributed to the heat I felt. I swept it upward into a ponytail. If, for some reason, I didn't get every hair up neat and tight, I redid it over and over until every hair was in place. This continued until my arms ached, yet I wouldn't give up this daily compulsion of perfection. I knew if I continued the process long enough, eventually, it would be flawless and I'd be satisfied.

If anyone wanted to discuss these issues or question my behavior, I put up a wall of resistance. The depths of my beliefs were deeply rooted. I felt my patterns and actions were necessary, and whether they were psychological or not didn't seem to matter. Advice was immediately rejected. I simply replied a new approach wouldn't work. I didn't think other people understood my behavior or suffering.

Living at home was very stressful for each and every one of us. I had been a free animal out in the wild, and now I felt confined. I didn't know where to turn or what to do with my life. The sponge bathing was not enough to keep me cool. The only thing that seemed to work was to be motionless in bed. As soon as I exerted myself, I was too hot to eat. This left out preparing meals, going up and down stairs, or even walking down the hallway. I didn't have a formula that worked; I was scared to move. My father was a firm believer in taking a person's body temperature when he or she felt ill. That was sufficient in terms of diagnosing an illness. Mine read normal.

When it was mealtime, I occupied the upstairs bathroom for a sponge bath in cold water. Even that made me nervous, as if I was under observation. I was afraid a family member was outside the door, waiting to use the bathroom and wondering why I was taking so long. That fear added extra warmth to the heat I already experienced. When I finally finished bathing, I was very demanding and impatient. I needed my food in front of me as quickly as possible, before I was hot all over again.

With the least amount of moving around possible, I called my mother and said, "Okay, I'm ready to eat."

My mother brought my meals upstairs, and she took the tray back down to the kitchen when I was finished. This went on for several days until my father became more and more impatient. Most anyone would say, "It's easy. Just sit down and eat." For most anyone else, it would be.

As long as I was warm, and the room felt warm, I could not bring myself to consume much food. A bite here and there was not healthy nutrition.

I was torn between feeling bad about my mother having to go up and down the stairs all the time and being afraid to go down to the kitchen without overheating. After many days of deliberation, I left the bedroom, washed up in cool water, and walked down the stairs. What I planned to eat, when I was upstairs, quickly changed when I entered the kitchen. I didn't care if I ate at all. I fought with myself over wanting to eat and not being able to eat. That, in turn, created a great amount of mental turmoil and frustration.

I knew I had to eat, but as soon as I ate, my body was hot. Then I had to walk outside. When I came back in, I was warmer than before I went out.

The same old story — nothing had changed. I knew I couldn't go back to the swimming. I had to come up with other options.

I heard rumors of an old inn being transformed into a health spa on the other side of town. I knew that no matter where I chose to live, my habits would follow me. The best I could hope for was having my own bathroom — a room where I was in control of the temperature and a place to hide when it was time to eat. I desperately needed a change of some sort. I talked to the owner. He said I could help out in the kitchen and serve meals, in exchange for a room at his spa, and be company for the girls that came there from New York City. The clientele reserved this place for fasting and for relaxing. Once the fasting was over, a very healthy diet was served. The spa brochure made it sound very appealing; little did anyone know what the building really looked like. It was a run-down, old place with possibilities, but the owner had very little money for improvements. Everyone was friendly and happy most of the time; it was the best I could hope for in my circumstances.

The owner was the only male there. I think he had things on his mind other than the sole position of proprietor. He asked me to join him in his bedroom one night. He said it was just to talk. The naive person that I was didn't realize he wanted more than conversation. I was shocked and educated at the same time. My sheltered life quickly changed. I left hastily. I had a thirst for interesting discussions when I wasn't bathing, but unfortunately, I didn't pick up on people's intentions.

This wasn't the best place to live, but I managed as long as the weather was cool. As soon as spring arrived, I was warm all the time, couldn't sit still, spent many sleepless nights, and was eating very little. The owner and his guests went to a nearby park to swim, but I couldn't afford the temptation. I was afraid one swim might draw me back into my old habits.

The heat became unbearable. I became weak and undernourished. My energy was depleted, and I was unable to comprehend what was going on around me. The owner of the spa called the ambulance, and I was transported to the nearest hospital, which was in Hudson.

During my hospital stay, nothing was resolved, discovered, or fixed. Before I was released, a social worker came into my room for a brief visit. She asked a lot of questions and, upon leaving, gave me her business card for future reference if needed. My mother drove me home from the hospital — another awkward and tense trip.

Chapter 10
House to House

I became a woman I did not know. It was obvious my parents were sad and helpless; all they saw was their daughter going down a path that lead nowhere. Needless to say, we were very frustrated and worn out. We tried living with each other, but it just didn't work. My habits and obsessions did not correspond with their lives, and they couldn't cope with my illness, issues, or whatever went on in my life at this time. I knew they struggled with the decision of asking me to leave. This whole situation wasn't easy on any of us.

Dad sat alone many times late at night, trying to make sense of it all. Some evenings he, my sister, and I sat around the kitchen table, looking for a solution. I was confronted with questions I didn't have the answers to. I had gone so far *off the track* that I didn't know how to be the daughter he once knew. At one time, my dreams were what his dreams were: healthy, happy, working woman, living a normal life. All of that was lost in a mired situation.

He didn't know what was going on or how I ended up in such a state. I didn't either. My parents exhausted all their avenues in an attempt to help me and couldn't continue. They even tried placing me in a rehabilitation psychiatric center in Connecticut. I went to the interview, and the director said I wasn't bad enough to be admitted. He didn't have any suggestions. I knew the trip was a waste of time long before I agreed to go; I only wanted to appease my parents. In fact, I didn't give them an immediate answer about going. The appointment at the center was just after lunch, and the mere thought of how I would go about a lunch in a strange environment frightened me. I knew if I didn't eat, I would develop a horrible migraine. I convinced myself, somehow, I could do this. I wouldn't think of eating a meal in a restaurant, so I brought a lunch, something simple and easy to eat quickly. It consisted of a hard-boiled egg, one slice of bread, an apple, and a diet drink. I felt this was a safe choice where I wouldn't become too overheated. I told my parents I wanted to eat alone. I chose a shady spot under a tree and sat there nervously, doing my best to get some nutrition into my stomach. I was so out of my own element, it was ridiculous to even think this setting could work. It was a day worth forgetting.

I was eating less and less. I envisioned a meal, and when I sat at the kitchen table to eat it, I became too warm. The headaches increased, I had chest pains, and I was weak. It wasn't long before I was back in the hospital, but only for one night. Again, the doctors didn't find anything abnormal. The social worker visited me once again. I wasn't sure where I was going to live next. I knew I couldn't live with my parents any longer. I was sure I made them miserable — and myself. It was a disheartening time for everyone I loved. Today, after some counseling from a very close friend, I have come to terms with the fact that leaving home was meant to be. What lay ahead was tough, but it was the only way I was going to heal. At the time I parted, I had no specific plans; maybe what was about to evolve was my destiny.

"Destiny is the bridge you build to the one you love."

I didn't know who *he* was, but destiny was out there somewhere. I wasn't looking for him at this time, yet when I look back to these days, I believe God was carrying me to him.

July 1978
Cold shower once a day
(plus a cold bath when available)

I agreed to go with the social worker. We traveled to a private home outside the city of Hudson. The home took in girls with *issues* and women who had no other place to go. My behavior was rather unique and in its own category. While there, I had no one to relate to, and I felt very alone.

It was the summer of 1978 — and a hot one. All the women with out of the ordinary problems stayed in the lower level of the house, which was a renovated basement. It was nice enough for what it was, if you liked being confined below ground, had no car, and waited for meals you could hardly eat. There was nothing to do all day but endure the miserable heat in the house or out in the yard. My new living arrangement was unbearable.

I knew there was a bathtub in the upper level of the house, and I devised a plan to cope with the heat. I set my alarm for five a.m. When it sounded, I quickly hit the shut-off button, so no one would wake. I went quietly up the stairs, knowing if one board creaked, I'd be caught. We were not allowed upstairs unless we were invited. I tiptoed to the bathroom, terrified as I took each step.

I managed a quick, cold bath and wished it could have lasted forever. I dried myself enough so I didn't drip water all over the floor, and hid any evidence of being there. I hurriedly went back downstairs and took a deep sigh of relief. Thank God, no one saw me.

I continued this same procedure a few more times until the woman of the house caught me. That was the end of the cold baths. And I received an extensive lecture.

The social worker arrived bright and early the next morning. She drove me to Albany, New York, where I had an interview with a doctor at a large, psychiatric center. I told the social worker I already went to one in Connecticut, and they wouldn't admit me. She still thought it was a good idea to keep the appointment. The doctor conducting the interview refused to admit me for the same reason: my condition didn't warrant admission into the facility. The day seemed longer than most, and it ended with a migraine. Between the trip and the home for girls, I wanted to scream. I thought to myself, "How could my predicament get any worse?"

One morning, I woke up hot from head to toe. I wasn't going to take another whole day overcome with heat. Frantic and in much despair, I went against the house rules. I turned the shower — on the lower level of the house — into a bathtub. I stayed in there so long that the water ran over the shower stall base and out onto the floor. You might say I flooded the place.

I was asked to vacate that afternoon.

The same social service worker came to the house and transported me to a new dwelling. It was another private home. The woman of the house used to take in people regularly but had stopped; however, she agreed to let me stay with her as a favor to the social worker.

In the beginning, it was great. The *nice lady* was there alone most of the time. Occasionally, her husband left New York City to spend time with his wife in the country. I gave her a brief synopsis of my life. I thought she genuinely cared. The social worker set me up for food stamps, which was barely enough for groceries. This *nice lady* purchased a variety of items I liked, especially fruit. She thought I might feel better eating foods with fewer calories and ones that produced less heat in my body.

Starting in August 1978, I took a cold bath once a day and a cold sponge bath three times a day.

I continued my water obsession. The *nice lady* didn't seem to mind my odd behavior, and I felt more at ease and relaxed than I had in a long time. In the morning, I immersed myself in a bathtub of cold water. Next, I went into my room and swept my hair up into a ponytail, proceeded to dress, and then went downstairs for breakfast. The morning went rather well, unless I was delayed with my hair. I was obsessed with perfection. I still worked at getting every strand of hair in place. If it wasn't perfect, I was afraid I wouldn't be able to eat breakfast. Before lunch and dinner, I took a cold sponge bath in the downstairs bathroom sink. She never commented on how long it took me. I assumed we were getting along just fine.

I didn't have my own transportation, and the *nice lady* took me with her wherever she went — even to my appointments with social services and trips to the grocery store.

Her daughter was building a house down the street. It was a nice diversion away from my problems. When I wasn't putting all my energy into bathing and staying cool, I enjoyed talking with the workers and watching the progress. It was a nice feeling to be included in their family. They often invited me at mealtime, but I always declined. I had my own set procedure before each meal — bathe and then eat immediately — and I was very particular about what I ate. I wanted to let go of my fears and be normal, but my thoughts convinced me otherwise.

One afternoon, they were discussing flooring. They mentioned the name of a local furniture store, and the owner happened to be a high school classmate of mine. The *nice lady* invited me to go along on their buying trip. For a brief moment, I was taken back to my teenage years. All my habits and rituals were out of mind. All I wanted to do was see my friend again. I didn't want to tell her all about what happened to me. I just wanted to see her beautiful face and spend time with a friend.

She was kind enough to loan me her Cadillac, so I could drive back home to see my parents. And she gave me extra money for gas.

The visit was brief but pleasant. I asked to have my car back. Dad said he had to think about it. After a few days, I received a long, awaited call. It felt good to be driving my own car once again.

The *nice lady* and I were getting along great until her husband and son arrived one weekend. Once the weekend was over, the *nice lady* changed her attitude towards me. She was distant and unresponsive.

I was usually quite tuned into behavioral changes. Then my nerves responded accordingly. It didn't matter how much cold water I used, I still felt hot.

I overheard the *nice lady's* relatives talking about renovating another house, but it was at a standstill. I commented that I enjoyed makeovers, so they offered to give me a tour. The house was in walking distance.

I decided it would be a perfect, temporary place for me to eat my meals. It would alleviate the stress of eating with people I thought disapproved of my behavior. I could make it my own house, and no one would be the wiser. The plan was a good one, as long as I didn't get caught.

The house was cool and clean, and even had a ceiling fan. The sink and a large counter area were connected. This enabled me to sponge bathe and then quickly eat. With this setup and solitude, I ate a lot more food. And the fact that no one was around to watch this unorthodox routine left me feeling guilt free. I wasn't being watched and judged as a weird, crazy person. I was happy in my own little world. For the first time in years, I looked forward to eating. I really enjoyed every mouthful. It was paradise.

I heard the family talking about someone being in the house uninvited and what they would do if that someone got caught. I knew right away my paradise was over. Soon after, I got the cold shoulder. Perhaps they expected a confession from me, but I was too embarrassed and remained mute. Even if I told her relatives why, no one would have understood. And I was afraid the *nice lady* would ask me to leave her house. I continued to deceive them for a little while longer until I sensed way too much danger. From then on, I returned to the *nice lady's* house for all my bathing.

It was around five thirty on a Saturday morning, the house was quiet, and all were asleep, including me. With no warning whatsoever, my door flew open. I awoke to the presence of the *nice lady* standing in my doorway. I thought maybe someone was hurt, or the house was on fire, or some other disaster occurred. Morning was not my best time. It always took me about thirty minutes to wake up as I made an attempt to adjust to the temperatures around me. I definitely didn't expect someone talking to me from the entrance to my bedroom. I preferred to be mute until after I took a long, cold bath and ate my breakfast.

I heard a voice say, "I want you out of here after breakfast."

I was stunned. The *nice lady* wasn't nice anymore, and why? I kept asking her why. What did I do? Can't you tell me? I thought you liked me.

The odd thing was, I assumed we were pals. It was a long time since I found someone to confide my feelings. I thought she understood my need to stay cool overshadowed every aspect of my life. No matter how much I pleaded with the *not so nice lady*, she wouldn't change her mind.

I was naive and didn't realize that what she did as a favor to social services did not necessarily mean her behavior toward me personally was any more than simple courtesy. When she demanded I leave the house, I was shocked. My mind was unable to comprehend this part of my journey. I thought, "How do people treat other people like this?"

While I was trying to eat some breakfast, in between the tears, she dropped the bomb. She accused me of taking money from a mug in the kitchen closet. I had no idea what she was talking about. I told her I would never do something like that. It was useless talking to this *not so nice lady*. Her mind was made up, and I think her husband and son played a very big role in her assessment.

Although her husband had some gambling issues, I was the likely culprit for her accusations. I thought her son liked me, and I asked him to tell his mother I wouldn't do such a thing; but they were family, and ultimately, I was not.

I packed the few things, and on my way out the door, I begged *the not so nice lady* to change her mind. She closed the door in my face. That was the last time I ever saw her.

"Be kind whenever possible. It is always possible."

"Our prime purpose in this life is to help others.
And if you can't help them, at least don't hurt them."
Dalai Lama

I remembered what a friend told me, "The only person you can count on is yourself." I felt rather whittled down as I stood on her doorstep. I had to leave the property, and the question was: where to next?

On a previous visit, her son gave me his telephone number. He said to call if I ever needed help. I certainly seemed to need it now, even though I wasn't sure I wanted help from him. I was afraid to call him, but I thought it was my only option, given I had nowhere else to go.

I called from a nearby telephone booth, and he told me to come over. It was way out of town on some winding back road. I was upset from his mother's recent verbal attack and extremely nervous around her son. Cold water wouldn't have helped me eat because of the state I was in. And I was too scared to even think about going through my water ritual; therefore, I didn't eat any dinner. We talked very little, and then he made some advances. His reason for offering help was not unselfish at all.

I quickly told him I wasn't interested. I only needed a place to crash for one night. He became very arrogant and nasty. He informed me that I had to be out of his house early the next day. I would have left right then, but it was too late, and I was afraid I'd get lost.

First thing in the morning, before the sun made its debut, I was on my feet and ready to leave. I gathered my belongings and couldn't get out of his house fast enough. He came out the door yelling obscenities and calling me the worst names I ever heard. I was mortified, but fortunately, nothing more happened.

Again, I had nowhere to go. I contacted the woman at social services. She made arrangements with a local motel and emphasized it would only be a month. I thought I was lonely before. But this was far worse. I knew absolutely no one except my friend at the furniture store. She had a business to run; I couldn't just stop in and talk with her at any given time.

I had too much spare time, and that only intensified my dismal situation. There was a diner within walking distance of the motel, and it was open twenty-four hours a day. I never ate there, but I ordered a beverage I didn't drink. Ordering something allowed me to sit for a while. I was hungry, but the fear of becoming too warm hovered over me as if it were the devil himself testing me. I was afraid to eat. I brought food back to my motel room; however, the scene didn't change. I was reluctant to eat there as well. As soon as I thought about eating, my body turned warm, and then I became anxious about putting food into my mouth.

If I ate and my head became extremely hot, how could I go to sleep? How could I get rid of the heat? The tap water wasn't cold at all. In order to make water feel cold, one has to put ice in it. That was my answer to this dilemma. I decided to fill the tub with water and add ice. The motel had plenty, and they even supplied a bucket. How convenient was that? The ice supply disappeared each day. The motel manager came to me and asked why I needed so much ice. He said it was a complimentary item, but for a minimal amount — not to empty the bin each day.

I sat in the lobby of the motel to pass the time and eagerly anticipated a little communication with the motel owner. He was not much of a conversationalist. I was lonely, so I walked to the diner in search of someone to talk to, but none of the strangers there cared to talk either. The days dragged on, and on, and on; I could have sworn each day was longer than twenty-four hours.

As the end of the month grew closer, my high school friend found me another place to live temporarily. This was good news and bad news. The home was way out of town. I had no clue as to what my environment would be. This made my decision difficult. The person I was going to stay with offered to pick me up after she finished work. Even as I sat in her car, late in the evening, I still wasn't sure if this was the right decision. I didn't know if I could manage to eat in her home, but I finally gave in and said yes. She drove for what seemed to be hours, and we arrived at a tiny trailer. The size alone worried me.

I became claustrophobic as soon as I stepped into the first room, and it felt like an oven; it was so hot. My stomach was in a knot, and there was fear written all over my face. I knew I could not stay there. I told her as much, and that didn't make her happy. She worked all day, drove all this way late at night, and now I told her I couldn't stay. She took me back to the motel at one o'clock in the morning.

The summer of 1978 was fading out, and the early signs of autumn approached. At the end of the month, social service stopped paying the rent. My time was up. I begged the motel owner to let me stay longer. He gave in to a couple more days, but then I had to leave. I put a few items in a paper bag and sat in my car for a moment, pondering where to next.

I felt as if my options had run out, and I had boarded a train to *Nowhereville*.

Chapter 11
Angel on Earth

I knew that sitting in the parking lot wasn't going to solve my problems; I had to drive somewhere. I had not returned to Albany, New York since the social worker took me to the interview at the psychiatric center. For some unknown reason, I was drawn to that city on this departure day, in September 1978.

My neighbor in Colorado was originally from Albany. She had since moved back into the area and was the only person I knew. I looked through the local telephone book and found her number and address. It was so good to hear her voice on the other end of the line. I told her my predicament. She clarified the directions, and it wasn't long before I was sitting in her living room. She was happy to see me; and I was overjoyed to see her. We chatted until the day went into darkness. Then she offered me her couch, which I gladly accepted. I ended up staying with her for about a month.

Cold bath once a day

Bathing in cold water was still part of my morning ritual. I eliminated the ice in my bath; I didn't want her to notice I had resorted to this behavior and acquired an addiction. I tried to get in and out of the bathroom before anyone else was up. My plan didn't always work, and I held up the household for a considerable amount of time. My friend was extremely patient and always made me feel right at home. I was supposed to be looking for quarters of my own, but there was always something wrong with the prospective housing.

I knew I was overstaying my welcome. It wasn't right, leaning on a friend for so long without any prospects in sight. She gave me *shelter from the storm* and time to catch my breath. One beautiful, autumn day in 1978, I departed, with no idea of where I was going.

This wonderful woman was my bridge to finding the man of my dreams
and a future of optimism and happiness.

I drove up and down the streets of downtown Albany. Finally, I stopped and purchased a newspaper. I looked at a few run-down apartments in an intimidating and creepy section of the city. I quickly left that neighborhood.

Then I scanned Rooms For Rent. There was one ad that looked like a possibility. It was around seven o'clock in the evening when I dialed the number. A man answered, and his voice was pleasant. I didn't know it at the time, but a guardian angel was coming into my life.

It was dark, but I didn't get lost. The house was small but appealing. There were many trees across the road, which gave it a little bit of a country feeling. I rang the doorbell, feeling hopeful. The owner answered the door, and there was something about him I liked. He was a nice-looking man, relatively shorter than I, and his name was Paul. He invited me inside; we sat in the kitchen and talked for a bit. In only a few minutes of conversation, I knew he cared and sincerely wanted to help me. He worked in construction and was separated from his wife. He wanted someone home when he was working, plus having roomers would add to his income.

The house was a split-level. It had three bedrooms upstairs and one very big bedroom below the main floor. I mentally listed all my needs with question marks.

Would the room be big enough (small created a warm feeling)?
Would the room be cold enough to sleep in?
Would I be able to bathe in ice water?
How will I get all the ice I need?
Would I have enough time to bathe in cold water?
When I eat my meals, will the kitchen be cold enough?
Will the owner of the house allow all of this?

The questions, doubts, and fears shifted around in my head endlessly. I knew once I made up my mind to stay, I wouldn't have any control over the temperatures of the house. That made me very nervous.

Paul and I went from room to room. I felt like Goldilocks and the Three Bears. I sat on the bed in one room, then the next, and so on. I wandered in and out of the three rooms, sizing each one up. Then I repeated this process over and over again. I was anxious and not sure if the house would be cold enough for me to manage.

I sat in Paul's kitchen on the evening of October 20, 1978. I couldn't make up my mind if I was staying or leaving. The odd thing was, I had nowhere else to go. When I thought about it many years later, I wondered what the big decision was under the circumstances.

I had less than five dollars in my pocket. Along with that, I possessed one bad apple, a small amount of apple juice, and a raw egg.

Other than the clothes on my back, I had a few garments in a paper bag. I was wearing one of my favorite dresses, the old standby: a handmade, polka-dotted sundress my mother made; the same well-worn sandals from years ago; and a shabby, thin raincoat over my dress.

I finally made my decision to stay. Paul told me not to worry about the rent at this time.

What I didn't know then was that God brought me to this man, this angel, and to this very house where I would find peace, total unconditional love, and many new beginnings. Those, in turn, would lead me to become a happy, healthy person — from one who had definitely lost her way.

During this time, in 1978,
I began taking cold showers with ice in the bathtub three times a day.

I was not a person to change easily. I couldn't. My daily obsessive-compulsive behavior produced the results I needed to survive. I was nervous about asking my landlord for extra ice. I figured I might as well be upfront and truthful right from the beginning. I told him I used ice every day when I showered; it was a necessity for my survival. He wanted to know why. I told him of my heat intolerance. This unusual request wasn't a problem. Whenever I needed ice, day or night, Paul went to the store. I didn't know it yet; but the wonderful part of this new environment was Paul's patience, kindness, an attempt to understand, and his unlimited time. Paul gave me time. I don't mean an hour or two, but years and years to slowly heal.

I was a big disruption in my landlord's life. His daily routine drastically changed. He had more worry and stress. Each day brought unexpected moments. He didn't have any medical experience or knowledge about my condition. He relied on his common sense, and he never gave up on me. Paul believed I did what I had to do in order to survive. And for the most part, he wasn't going to question it.

My inner struggles and unanswered questions lingered. The thoughts in my head raced around and around: why me, what is happening, and why? I just wanted to sit at a table and eat, or walk into any room without the intense, overpowering heat. Why did I have this need to cool my skin?

At the time, I didn't look to God for the answers. I only thought about my discomfort and tried to deal with it on my own. Later on, I realized God was looking after me; there is no other feasible way I could have survived and made my way to Albany.

Christ said, "You must lose your life to gain it."

I had just about lost it several times. Possibly, my new home would be a turning point in my life.

I never heard of the poem "Footsteps" until several years after moving into Paul's home. I knew when I read it that the poem was talking to me. This poem is one of my favorites. Even though I grew up attending church on Sundays, I didn't know much about the Bible. I believed in God and His love but never thought about Him too much while I was in this water-addiction dilemma. I believe prayer requires a certain amount of mental concentration. My mental power was directed elsewhere, so it was impossible to focus on the spiritual. When I was living at home, a friend/pediatrician tried to bring me to the Lord. She introduced me to a group of young people that belonged to The Way®, a nondenominational Biblical research, teaching, and fellowship ministry. I think she knew I was in trouble. This was her small but powerful way of trying to help. It gave me the opportunity to attend some church services and social gatherings. The believers prayed I would find the Lord. I went a few times, eagerly waiting for a miracle to happen.

I thought, "If only God would heal me."

After the initial asking, my mind was elsewhere. I tried to be enthusiastic. But the warmth I was feeling became the winning force. The problems I had with environmental challenges made it very difficult to interact with anyone. I was only able to cope with the temperature in the building for a short time. Within that time frame, I wanted a "quick fix." And because it didn't happen, I quickly drifted away from these good people. Many years later, I learned patience is a virtue when waiting for God. Our time, as opposed to God's time, isn't the same. However, I strongly believe that as I was stumbling and trying to stay afloat, He was carrying me. I just didn't realize it. For without Him, I am sure I would have perished. I now believe He had a plan.

If this book helps even one person, then I, along with my experience and the book, have become instruments of God.

Money, and where it was going to come from, should have been a worry, but it wasn't. I believe people were placed in my path at just the right time. Some were strangers, and others I knew. Somehow, from one moment to the next, the little cash I possessed carried me through. God didn't make it easy, but I believe that was part of the healing process. For example, I had only a few dollars when I knocked on Paul's door; however, he put the rent money on hold until I was able to pay him.

Years later, and even to this day, Paul jokingly says, "And she still owes me the first month's rent!"

Paul wasn't a rich man. He worked when there was a construction job. When the job ended, he was laid off. Then he sat in union hall every day until he was called for the next job. Paul paid for everything even though he couldn't always count on the next paycheck. He bought all the ice I needed, and that was definitely an unexpected item on a minimal paycheck. The refrigerator was well stocked, the house was always warm — too warm, and his bills were always paid on time. He didn't complain about the amount of water I used. He never asked me to contribute any money toward maintaining the house or the car.

When Paul and I reminisce about these times, he comments, "There was something very different about our relationship back then. We had a stronger connection; we needed each other more."

Materialistic things weren't important. Our needs were much different, a day-to-day survival. We didn't have the money for one thing, but I think it was good we didn't. We appreciated the space around us instead of accumulating *stuff* we didn't need.

The space enabled Paul and I to think about each other and not be distracted by an object having more importance than the two of us. In between the fears and the struggles, we enjoyed the things that are readily available: the sweet smell of fresh air, a sunset, wildflowers, a great song on the radio, a smile, a hug, and, most of all, the power that brought us together. I bought the newspaper just in time to see Paul's ad under *Room for Rent*. I didn't search the ads for months; sometimes the best things show up with the least amount of effort.

Unpaid hospital bills from the past were sent to me and to my father. Paul had a minimal amount of education, but he knew I had to file for bankruptcy. I didn't have any money. That meant I couldn't get a credit card for several years. Paul's mind was always thinking. He was alert, and he listened. With no time to waste, and as soon as it was possible, he assured I would have a credit card in my name.

Paul couldn't believe I wasn't on welfare before I arrived at his house. He said my medical bills would have been taken care of, and I could have had food stamps. He later found out I didn't qualify for welfare because of my last name. At the time when I was told I didn't qualify, I left it at that. I was too timid to pursue it any further.

Paul took me to social services, in Albany, to apply. What fun that was. Trying to get me to sit still in a warm building was like stopping an ice cream cone from dripping in the sun. It was a struggle, to say the least. All the years that I lived in a cold environment, I hardly ever had a headache; but now living more and more indoors, I had headaches with increasing regularity. Becoming overheated, plus getting a headache, equals "Let me out of here."

The extended visit to the social service office made me physically miserable. By the time we left, neither of us was to be reckoned with.

Chapter 12
Ice Cubes, Ice water

The pattern I developed at the motel resurfaced here with Paul's compliance and access to a freezer. I started taking ice baths again, and Paul kept the freezer well stocked; in fact, that compartment consisted mostly of ice. Paul routinely asked if I had enough ice. Sometimes one store ran out, so he went to another. When I first arrived, I used one bag in the bathtub. As time passed, I used many more until I made it unbelievably cold. Paul was buying, at least, twenty-one bags of ice a week. I didn't realize how dangerous the ice was to my health. I was probably numbing my brain and lowering my body temperature instantaneously.

Any appointments during the day were stressful. It didn't matter if I was indoors or outdoors. On sunny days, the car felt like a sauna. The sun and warmth of the day, plus the confinement, didn't blend well together. My body accumulated more heat than it could tolerate. Paul looked for a doctor with evening hours, preferably after seven o'clock. He finally found one not too far from the house.

We were almost to the doctor's office when I told Paul I was too hot. Without hesitation or any irritating questions, he turned the car around and drove home. We didn't reschedule the appointment. I liked gloomy, rainy, dreary, dismal days the best. I didn't have to contend with the sun's rays and sweltering heat. When I entered a building, there wasn't such a drastic temperature change. I seemed to function in reverse of the general population.

Whenever we had an overcast day, Paul said, "This is your kind of day, a Munster Day." He brought a smile to my face with his terminology. He came out with funny, unexpected phrases, and the more I thought about them, especially later on, I laughed all over again.

Paul believed it was important I have a doctor. A new, health park opened, and it was only five minutes from our door. Luckily, Paul was eligible, because it was offered through his union. We weren't married, but somehow, I was accepted. Paul wanted me to have a variety of care, including dental. He thought this medical group would be perfect, because we didn't have to travel too far. I never liked leaving the house early. Most of the time, the doctors weren't on schedule. I wanted to walk in, sit down, and be seen. If I had to wait more than ten minutes, the room became too warm. I found it difficult to be still, so I paced back and forth. This continued until

I couldn't take the wait. The end result: most appointments were close to impossible to keep. Paul was sure some doctor would find a drug to help me. He knew I needed help, but no one else was in his corner, not even me. None of the doctors appeared to be overly interested in something out of the ordinary. The only good part: I was on file with a general practitioner.

October was drawing to a close. I still wore a sundress and sandals, plus searching for cold. After the ice baths, I was only cold for a short time. By the time I reached the kitchen, I was warm. I didn't eat a sufficient amount, and I became undernourished. I still enjoyed a long walk in all kinds of weather. I was determined to wear lightweight clothing outdoors, no matter what the weather was. Unfortunately, the outdoor temperature was dropping, and so was mine. As soon as my feet hit the front stoop, Paul was securely positioned in a chair near the kitchen window. His eyes held fast to the cloudy glass, making sure I was in sight every few minutes. Tense with worry, he was relieved each time I passed but nervous because I stayed out there so long. He patiently waited and worried the whole time I was outdoors. His eyes never left the street, always checking to make sure I was still alive. That gave him some peace of mind.

When worrying got the best of him, he hollered out the door, "Is that your last lap? How about coming inside?"

When I finally came back in the house, I didn't want to talk to anyone or even think about eating. My skin didn't just tingle like most folks; I was burning up as if I had a fever. And it lasted until bedtime. As bad as I felt, I couldn't wait to get back outside.

I had forgotten all about *Big Bertha*, until a friend and I reminisced about this part of my journey. He didn't know me when I first rented a room from Paul. And when he read my story, he was amazed. All he remembered was seeing a strange, young girl walking past his house at night, in the dead of winter, wearing what looked like a long, fur coat.

Paul would have loved it if I had worn something so warm. It was difficult enough to get me into *any* heavy coat. Paul insisted I wear something that was warm, heavy, and long if I was determined to be out in the cold weather.

I didn't want to spend a lot of money on a coat I didn't want in the first place. I thought I found the bargain of the year when I purchased a wool coat in a local retail store for eighteen dollars. And it was a size eighteen, which meant it was big all over. The more room between the wool and me, the better. Paul thought it was too long and too big, so he called it *Big Bertha*. She served her purpose and put Paul's mind at ease during the cold, winter months. She even rode in the trunk of my car many years later because Paul insisted I have an emergency coat with me, in case my car broke down.

Paul watched a young girl in trouble. He wanted to help *fix* the problem, yet he didn't know what to do. He called my father for assistance. Dad didn't have any ideas and told Paul he should consider calling the police. He didn't want anything to do with me. When I lived with my family, all the doctors' reports showed nothing, and Dad felt it was a waste of time. I think he was convinced it was psychiatric.

At this particular point in time, I was so engrossed in keeping my body cool that I was oblivious to anyone's remarks. I didn't care who said what.

Years later, when Paul commented on my father's remark, I wasn't upset. My parents just didn't know. If I were in their shoes, I might have replied with a similar answer. I put a lot of stress on my family. I certainly wasn't an easy person to live with.

My parents were more than fair. They tried to help in any way they could so I was able to continue my lifestyle. I did what I did in order to function, even though I was destroying myself in the process. I thought I knew what was right for me at the time. Anyone taking a good look could see otherwise.

Paul's house was sufficiently warm; however, I did everything in my power to keep my body dangerously cold. I wasn't ingesting enough calories, and even if I was, the ice water was the predominant factor in this scenario.

Paul knew he had to do something and prayed it was the right thing. He made all the decisions because I wasn't capable. He took my body temperature, and it was plummeting. He called our doctor at the health park, but he wasn't in at the time. Paul spoke with the doctor on call and told him my body temperature was dangerously low. Paul didn't know what to do. The staff didn't take him seriously, probably because they never encountered a similar situation before this telephone call. Paul was now in a place where he had to make some very strong decisions, which could either kill me or keep me alive. He was alone in this mess.

He went with his common sense. He told me I had to take a hot bath. I pleaded and begged: no hot bath. He insisted, and after much debate, I gave in. The water did bring up my temperature. It was temporary because there wasn't enough *fuel in the furnace*, so to speak.

After the bath, I was very sleepy and weak, and I went to bed. I asked Paul to keep the shades down for total darkness. I only wanted rest and to sleep. I recall seeing two strangers in my bedroom, and they asked me questions I didn't comprehend. They were there and then not there. I didn't know if I were in a dream state or a real movie about my life. I insisted on the room remaining dark as long as I was alone. The light hurt my eyes, and when anyone turned a light on, I couldn't wait for the darkness again. They wanted me to sit up while they questioned me, but I could barely hold my head up. All I wanted to do was go to sleep. My head was heavy. It was as if someone or something continuously closed my eyes for me. No matter how hard I tried to keep them open, my eyelids would shut.

After the strangers, who were social workers, left my room, I slept some more. Paul allowed it for a couple of days, but by then, I wasn't eating. He decided to bring me down into the living room and nearer to the kitchen; possibly, the smells from the kitchen would entice me to eat something. I lay there day and night, only getting up to use the bathroom.

Christmas was approaching. Paul attempted to cheer me up. He played Christmas music all day long and set up a small, artificial, Christmas tree with tiny, white lights. He placed it on the hi-fi so I could see it when I opened my eyes. I remember dozing and seeing the blurry lights from time to time when I opened my eyes.

I had no idea of the danger I was in. I was tired out from years of punishing my body. It was almost as if my body went into hibernation to protect itself from any more harm.

After lying there for several days, I was delirious and spacey. I began to see rabbits, cats, and birds floating all around the room. Paul told me later on I was hallucinating. All I wanted to do was sleep on the couch forever. I didn't even want to move into another room. Paul encouraged me to sit at the kitchen table. I couldn't keep my head up long enough without my entire body falling over. He tried to tolerate all my choices until they became undoubtedly questionable; then he had to intervene. He took my body temperature from time to time, and when the thermometer read ninety-two degrees, he knew I was in danger. He told me we were going to the hospital. I made a strong statement, trying to convince him to let me stay at home.

"I don't want to go to any hospital. Please, don't take me there," I pleaded.

He wouldn't hear of it. Paul, as short as he was, picked me up and carried me to his car.

I was barely coherent. Yet during these dangerous times when my life was hanging in the balance, I never thought I was that bad off or in any real danger. I kept plugging along. I felt there would always be a tomorrow. Somehow, deep down in my soul, I knew I would live. I never thought about dying from low, body temperature.

I must have left this world for a short time, because I didn't remember the ride to the hospital or the entrance to the ER. When I opened my eyes the next morning, I was in the psychiatric ward at Albany Medical Center; I was moved from one hospital to another during what I called an *outer-body experience*. The only thing I recalled was *floating around in outer space*. I was holding on to the moon. I didn't want to drift out into nothingness. The amount of space around me was black, vast, and endless. I was terrified my grip wasn't strong enough, and at some point, the strength in my fingers might fail me. If that happened, the end was near.

For the first time, I was afraid. And I kept repeating the same thing, "I don't want to die. I want to go back to Earth. I don't want to die, and I want to go back to Earth." There were other people out there with me, none of whom I recognized. I wanted to hug someone, but no one was close to me — only the moon. My arms were strong, and I was able to hold on to the big, massive moon the entire time. I had a weird sensation that if I let go of the moon, maybe I wouldn't see Earth.

I always thought the heavens were gorgeous on a moonlit night. During my absence — when I was dangling from the moon, and space was consumed with a dark, unattractive, eerie force — it wasn't quite the same.

I told Paul about my experience. His comments were few, but he said he was glad to have me back.

Many years later, I received a book as a gift, *The Case for Heaven* by Mally Cox-Chapman. The book was excellent, and after reading it, I thought I might have had a near-death experience. I wrote the author a letter, telling her about what happened to me. She was quite confident I experienced an NDE. It was rather unique to add this to my life's journey; however, I think I shall pass on another one.

I felt rested, peaceful and hungry. I wasn't too warm or frantically trying to remedy that feeling. I had acquired a new freedom; I wasn't thinking about ice cubes and ice water. It was as if someone whispered in my ear and said, "You are now entering a positive sector in your journey."

There were two nurses fussing over me. Blessed with kind voices, and happy souls, they were pleasant to be around. I felt safe whenever they were near. Joy filled the air each time they came in to check on me. On the first day, the nurses helped me sit up and served me a breakfast of scrambled eggs, toast, orange juice, and tea. I savored every mouthful as if I had never eaten scrambled eggs before. It tasted wonderful.

When I was admitted into the hospital, my body weight was a little over one hundred pounds. My body temperature was a low eighty-eight degrees. Upon hearing this, Paul bought new thermometers, because ours only registered ninety-two degrees. There wasn't a one in the Capital District. After eliminating pharmacy after pharmacy, he finally found one in downtown Albany. He special-ordered a dozen.

Paul knew I was ill and prayed a good doctor would listen to our plea. Dr.

Lyn Howard, the top nutritionist at Albany Medical Center, became interested in my case and took me on as a patient. After being in the psychiatric ward for about a week, she transferred me to the main hospital. Dr. Howard specialized in eating disorders, and my medical history certainly indicted one. The very low body temperature attracted her as well. As she began looking further into my history and my actions, the question was: What came first, the chicken or the egg? In the beginning, did I do something to create my low body temperature, or did I have a condition that caused the feeling of heat, which led me to cold water and caused the drop in body temperature?

Dr. Howard inserted a feeding tube, which added extra nutrition to my daily diet. She and her team hoped both the tube and the eating would give my body the boost it needed to return to normal. After much observation, she believed it was also my goal to do everything possible in order to eat. The term for the diagnosis could still be the same, but the underlying cause could be different. At this point, it wasn't psychiatric; it was mostly medical, which eased my mind considerably. Now the work would begin: getting back into the real world.

Every day for the next few months, the nurses weighed me several times throughout the day. Vials of blood were drawn. My temperature was documented. They wrote down what I ate and required many twenty-four-hour urine tests. Plus there were machines by my bed, recording pertinent information.

I was in the hospital during the Christmas holiday. I remember a rather dull-lit room, with dreary, colorless walls, and the low thud and clunk of the heating system. It was a day of nothing, except to wait, vitals every so often, and then a meal. Late in the afternoon, Paul came into my room, carrying a miniature, Christmas tree with lights and tiny ornaments. As he entered my room, the atmosphere changed. He was smiling from ear to ear. I could see he was anticipating my reaction. Without a doubt, I was blessed to have a compassionate man in my life. He and Dr. Howard managed to get the tree lights turned on, too!

Paul never missed a day of visiting me at the hospital. He brought me flowers and cards and, on some days, a tiny gift — jewelry — to cheer me up. He brought exotic fruit: mangos, avocados, dates, figs, melons, and dried fruit. Anything he could think of that might taste good and get me to put on a few pounds.

I had a wonderful surprise when my sister came for a visit and brought me a tiny, Christmas tree. It was some time since I saw any of my family — Paul and I were our own family — distant from everyone. It meant a lot to see her standing in my hospital room. She made a special trip just to be with me.

When I was admitted into the hospital, my hair was quite long. It was quite disheveled after all my time in bed and lack of care. The attending nurse washed it, put it in tight braids, and neatly piled it on top of my head. My hair was away from my face and out of my neck. The new look and how I felt contributed to a feeling of coolness. Plus it helped me emotionally. I was transformed into someone different than the person I knew in the past, at least on the outside.

From this time forth, whatever gave me a little more out of life, I held on to it. The new hairstyle was one of those things. I wouldn't accept having my hair hang down anymore. As soon as it was washed, it had to be braided exactly like the nurse did it. This caused more stress than you can imagine, just finding someone to braid it the exact same way.

On some issues — like this one, for example — many people questioned if my reasons were psychiatric or medical. Paul never did. Whatever helped me get through the day, he went along with, although sometimes a good fixation became a bad obsession.

From November 1978 to July 1979, I took a warm sponge bath once a day. There were no showers or regular baths.

For seven years, I put my body through quite an ordeal. I was physically depleted and worn out. My senses were dull, emotions were minimal, and I didn't even have any passion left. The illness took over my life. All I cared about was being cold. That was all I knew. I could only hope my body would never be so deteriorated again. I needed extensive rest, which the hospital provided. Most days, in between the testing, I slept. I didn't exert myself. I ate moderately; thus, I was able to stay relatively cool. I was managing with a warm sponge bath instead of my ice baths, at least for now.

When my hospital stay was about to end, I was tense. I was adapted to the hospital environment and wasn't sure what would happen when I returned home. Would the addiction return? What would I do all day? I was quite content in the hospital. I had a new life here and liked it. The need to bathe in cold water was gone. I had a lot of people to interact with, whereas before, I was in my own sad world.

But I didn't have much of a choice about staying or leaving. In a very short time, I would be sleeping in my own bed. I was scared about the transition. The hospital was comfortable, it gave me some security, and the worries of the past were gone. Once I walked out of the hospital, my life would be different. Paul and I would soon be on our own without the doctors and nurses and a schedule to follow. Left to my own devices, I didn't trust myself. A nurse prepared my sponge bath water; would I use cooler water over time? Paul and I had great faith in Dr. Howard; if anyone could help us, she could. I felt remarkably better when she was near — as if she and the staff were saving my life.

Every day wasn't perfect, but the interaction l had with the staff put a new spin on my life; a fraction of something normal was starting to unfold — a taste of being around people again. I found it difficult to let go of this new existence.

Before being discharged, my doctor and I talked about having a home aide service come to the house. She felt I should have someone with me during the day until I regained my strength, especially when Paul was working. My needs were many at the time: assistance with chores, bathing and personal care, fix meals, make sure I was eating, and drive me to my doctor's appointments. The aide's presence might help with a gradual weight gain and boost my confidence. It was very important that I increase, or at least maintain, the weight I achieved in the hospital. It seemed I couldn't be trusted to eat sufficiently. Paul had to work long hours, and home aide was a good, temporary choice. I thought they were wonderful. They took the place of the nurses. I had someone to talk to and style my hair, which to me was more important than the eating. I felt I was taking in plenty of food, and I didn't need anyone monitoring me. The way I talked, it sounded as if I was eating a banquet; but in reality, I wasn't.

Follow-up appointments were scheduled. I saw Dr. Howard every month. Upon each visit, vitals were taken, many vials of blood drawn to make sure my thyroid was fine, and other levels — too many for me to remember — checked. Some of my symptoms pointed to problems with the thyroid, yet my readings were always perfect. The nurse asked that I turn around to be weighed. I couldn't figure out what that was about. It was a new procedure for patients with eating disorders. Evidently, not seeing the numbers proved to be helpful — *out of sight, out of mind.*

Over time, Dr. Howard and I saw each other every two months. As I progressed, the appointments were spaced farther apart. Each visit was extremely thorough. What I did in between was totally on me. She had no control over that. I often wondered if there were other similar cases to mine. There was talk of a woman in England, but she died; there weren't any records, so no one could make a comparison.

I had several home aides: from the very young to the more experienced, and from different and interesting backgrounds. I asked a lot of questions, probably too many, but I wanted a friend. The first aide was with me for several months. She fixed my meals, bathed me, and was a great companion. My favorite aide was more my age, and we bonded on the first day. She was fun to be around, and our conversation was never dull. And yes, she could braid hair just like I wanted it. Once a week, she washed my hair and neatly braided it. Each time, I asked her to start very close to my head and make the braid as tight as possible. The tighter she did it, the cooler I felt. A very weird assumption; however, I argued, over such a notion, until the cows came home. I was cooler, end of discussion. My hair began to recede on the right side of my head.. The sensible thing would be to discontinue this style; however, I was persistent in my request for tight braids.

I anticipated the sixth day of the week — the day prior to the braiding. I had more energy, talked non-stop, and felt prettier. I couldn't imagine my schedule being any different. I treated this aide like a friend. We bonded, or I bonded and became too attached to her. I was sure life would continue like this forever, not realizing the reality of it ending. She got another job, and I was terribly heartbroken.

I was convinced no one could braid hair like my favorite aide. Another gal was sent, and she didn't even want to try. I totally lost it and shamefully fell apart. The tears exploded naturally; I was a wreck. The house was turned upside down over hair. I had to find someone that could fix my hair just like the last home aide, or I wouldn't get through the day. I even called the agency and complained about the aide they sent. They agreed to send a different girl.

The hair ordeal drove Paul and me crazy. He couldn't understand it, but he went along with my theory of how it made me feel. I was very sincere. I was living the drama. My actions from day to day convinced him there was something to what I proclaimed.

Looking back, I think there was a mixture of both reality and fear. For a long time, I used the cold water to fix my problem with the heat I felt. Now, I was out on a limb. I could fall very easily. I adopted many ways to compensate for using cold water. If any were eliminated, I was devastated.

While I was in the hospital, I had lots of people around me while I ate my meals. Before being admitted, I didn't want to see anyone in the morning before breakfast. I insisted on eating alone. Once home, I couldn't eat breakfast without someone in the room with me. The aides were there for the first half of the day. Paul was with me for dinner.

The household tasks created more heat than I could tolerate, so Paul and the aides did everything.

Once we were home and situated, I knew what the main topic of conversation would be: Eat a sufficient amount of food and stay out of the hospital. I was sure another topic would also arise: taking a hot bath. I was petrified of getting into a bathtub of warm water. I did everything in my power to stay cool; I couldn't risk getting into hot water. I was progressing somewhat, and I was afraid a bath would be a setback. I needed to control my skin. The hot water wouldn't allow me to do that. Once hot, how could I reverse it? I prayed Paul wouldn't insist on a hot bath. Once in a while, he hinted to the fact, but I told him a lukewarm sponge bath was sufficient.

I promised to be a *good girl* and concentrate on eating. In the hospital, the food was prepared for me, and I wasn't concerned about becoming overheated. Any exertion prior to a meal turned off my appetite. If I did any cooking, I had to find a way to cool down. In the past, I bathed in ice water.

Paul said he would cook if that would help. We had the most fantastic meals. Talk about food — quantity, and quality — we had quite a spread. Paul prepared dinner, washed the dishes, cleaned the house, did the laundry, and shopped for groceries. He did it all, plus he worked as a laborer in construction.

Many times Paul said, "Whatever it takes to make you eat, I'm for it."

I seemed to be on his mind all the time. At the market, he purchased a variety of foods. His philosophy was: satisfy the taste buds, and a person will eat, yet not overeat. If you wait too long, the taste buds will be gone, and it takes a long time to bring them back. Generally, if nothing tastes good, you won't eat it. He read in a magazine, "If you want people to like your food, cook with a lot of salt, sugar, and oil." Paul prepared sweetbreads, veal, liver, beef, chicken and fish, vegetables, potatoes, and pasta and rice dishes. We were living it up with cheesecake, wine or beer, breads, and ice cream. Every meal was a feast and a variety to choose from. It was amazing.

Paul often remarked, "If there is anything you might want to try, I'll buy it."

I had starved my body of good nutrition for a long time. Everything Paul prepared was scrumptious. I felt as if we were back in time, sitting at a table adorned with lavish food, and he was the king, and I the queen. But really, there was too much to eat. After awhile, I found it difficult to sit still without, once again, overheating. I began looking for a way to cool down after a meal. On some evenings, we went to the mall, which was only about ten minutes from the house. While I was in motion, I was cooler. And I couldn't see my stomach. When I was terribly thin, my stomach was flat. Eating all these wonderful foods gave me a bulge, and when I sat down, it showed even more. I wanted to gain a few pounds, but not all in one spot! Too much weight gain made me nervous, and I certainly didn't want to take drastic measures to lose it. I made peace with myself by psychoanalyzing the eating process. "It's okay to overeat if I walk a lot afterward. If I don't, I'll become too fat." Paul was happy with the weight gain.

He said, "I like a big woman."

It might seem odd to say, considering all I put him through, but we were now becoming very close friends. I felt as if I had known him my entire life. I was never comfortable talking with a man. With Paul, all those feelings disappeared. I told him just about everything, good or bad. He treated me with kindness, respect, and consideration. He was too good to me, and he cared more about my welfare than I cared for myself.

Paul said, "When I come home from work, all I need to see is you standing at the front door with your nice, big smile. That is enough for me."

The relationship with my family was still strained. Paul believed it was important to have more contact with them. I looked healthier and was maintaining my weight. He wanted my parents to see the improvement.

We managed a few trips to Copake. "Down river," Paul called it. It took about eighty minutes to drive to my hometown. It was important for me to return, but that was where my addiction started, and I was hesitant. And I was afraid to get too far from our house. When I was in an unfamiliar environment, other than the hospital, I lost control of my surroundings. It was far from perfect there, but in my own way, I was beginning to manage with a step-by-step routine. I didn't have that anywhere else.

I knew I should make the trip, and I wanted to see my parents. Around this time, my mother was diagnosed with pancreatic cancer. That alone was an important reason to spend some time with her.

Paul also wanted the trip to include paying back the people who were kind enough to lend me money before I arrived at his house.

Paul made more of an effort on my appearance than his own. He believed it was important for me to make a good impression and show I was taking good care of myself by wearing clothes that were more appropriate for the time of year. Knowing I would be miserable in any heavy material, he suggested a medium-weight, polyester skirt and a blouse to match. He thought layering the garments would allow me to add or take away a garment as necessary, so he also purchased a lightweight sweater. While we were shopping, he spotted a leather coat. He insisted I try it on. I was concerned about the cost and not being able to wear the coat if it made me too warm. It did look fantastic. Paul convinced me to accept it along with leather boots, a warm angora hat, and gloves. Preparation was vital, as with anything important. A stronger woman is what he wanted the world to see. He was sure these items would also boost my self-esteem and confidence. Paul was pleased I looked so good. I think he was quite proud of where we were in our lives.

A few days prior to our trip, I tried out my new outfit. I walked out our front door and tripped. Unfortunately, I cut my chin on the slate edging surrounding our flowerbed. I needed stitches, which delayed the trip. As soon as I hit, I knew I disappointed Paul. The pain was nothing compared to letting him down. I was saddened that my triumphant return was ruined.

When we finally went to see my parents, it was definitely worth the trip. My mother was thin, but overall, she looked good to me. I was glad Paul persuaded me to visit my parents. I was nervous about their reception, but it went well. My mother really liked Paul. He promised her that he would always take care of her daughter. Paul kept his word most definitely.

My mother was in and out of the hospital several times. We saw her in two different hospitals, and the third trip was the last time I saw her alive. My mother passed away in 1979, nine months after I arrived at Paul's house. When I was told my mother died, I was unhappy, but because I was more concerned with my selfish survival I didn't react like I would have before my illness. At that time, when someone close to me passed away, my heart ached with deep pain, feeling as if someone ripped it from my body. I was extremely open then to emotions and feelings: especially sorrow and loss.

Unintentionally, I allowed my illness and addiction to take over my life and my brain. My illness put a detachment between my mother and I causing each of us to struggle in our own way. Therefore, no communication existed between us. I believe my brain was numb and unresponsive to many pertinent emotions. The guilt for that and my reaction to my mother's passing never went away.

I knew it was my responsibility to attend the funeral services, yet the fear of how I would get there took precedence. Also, my mind put up a mental block of not accepting her death. I planned on coming back to life with all its glory, and wanted her to be a part of it.

If Mom had passed ten years later, I would have reacted much differently. I would have cried my eyes out for days. My heart would have ached every time I thought of her. She gave me so many wonderful moments and endless memories. There isn't a day that goes by where I don't do something that is connected to my mother. She is a huge part of who I am today.

After my release from the hospital, I put myself in a cocoon. The hospital was a safe haven, and the temperatures were moderately even. When I came home, I tried to keep that same climate. Venturing out of that condition was very scary. Once I left the cocoon, coming back to it wasn't the same for me. Temperature changes meant I had to readjust each time I went from hot to cold, or cold to hot. This was not easy after using cold water as my tool for years. Now, the cold water was gone, and my body was being made to adjust on its own. It didn't happen quickly and sometimes not at all.

Eating all three meals on *my habitual time schedule* was also a factor. It never, ever changed. At each meal, I needed to compose myself, relax, and create a quiet, peaceful setting. I took on this procedure to keep the heat in my body under control. I made all my appointments to fit my schedule. At this stage of my recovery, eating three healthy meals, at a given time, was very important. Unfortunately, I didn't want anything to interfere with that, even if it was someone dying. I'm sure that sounds very selfish and cruel. I hoped the funeral service would be later in the afternoon. It wouldn't help the temperature changes; but it would give me time to eat my lunch, travel, and be back home in time for dinner.

It didn't happen that way. At this point in my life, I never planned an outing two days in a row. The wake was at seven in the evening. The funeral was the following day. I attended my mother's wake but not without difficulty. Since the time of the wake was after my last meal, Paul and I thought this was the better one to attend. There was another obstacle: as a rule, we didn't go out of the house after dinner. The evening was generally cooler, and that meant another temperature change. This trip was something out of the ordinary.

Prior to any excursion, I acted the scene out in great detail in my mind. This gave me some assurance as to whether I could manage it or not. But some fear always lingered in the back of my mind. I was able to keep myself relatively cool at home, but in another location and with all the stress, could I do it? For me, a strict schedule with as little temperature change as possible was my security. I think it helped to alleviate the fear of going back to cold water.

The cooler months helped lessen any thoughts of using cold water. As July rolled around, the rooms in the house felt smaller. The air became heavy. I felt too confined. The temperature surrounding my body felt sticky and warm. Clothing stuck to my body. Foods I ate in the cooler months were now making my body too hot.

It was too much to tolerate. I allowed my mind to slip back in time. Thoughts of cold water dominated my thinking.

I needed to eat immediately after I ate a meal, so the bathing had to take place in my bedroom. This was the only way to stay cool for any length of time. Bathing in a *kiddy pool* took place during the hot summer months of 1979. However, it came to an abrupt disheartening end one noon in August and left me drowning in my sorrows until I fell into a deep sleep.

Chapter 13
A New Day, a New Beginning, and Then

Every step I climbed away from the cold water and toward improvement, I replaced it with some other obsession. Some were okay — others were not.

Much to my surprise, when I opened my eyes the next morning, the day looked a little brighter. What flabbergasted me more was I slept great. The previous day was a terrifying one. But for now, I was relaxed in the comfort of my bed — without a care in the world. Those endless days of thinking about cold water were eliminated, and in its place, there was a sense of newness and peace. The sound of quiet was a long-awaited gift; my head was clear and rested. I hadn't experienced this delight in over ten years. My mind finally gave me a break; I felt harmonious with all my surroundings. I wasn't thinking about getting rid of the heat. I had to admit I was somewhat grateful for what Paul did the previous day. I certainly didn't think so at the time, but in less than twenty-four hours ago, a huge burden was taken away.

Eventually, the consumption of food was definitely going to come up in conversation. During this *beautiful, new moment*, I put that thought immediately out of my head. I was going to be consistent in what I promised myself. I was not going to use cold water as a means to eat. However, I would not eat without immersing myself in cold water. Allowing myself to slip backward wasn't an option. Unfortunately, there was no justification to this reasoning. I just didn't see it.

I enjoyed the newfound freedom with less stress. When it was time to eat, I would allow myself a drink made of ice water, artificial sweetener, and a piece of fresh lemon. This concoction didn't contain any calories plus I added ice, an assurance my body would stay cool. And it would look as if I were eating something.

Before I put one foot on the floor, I knew I wanted this day to be unique for the both of us. What about a nice drive up to Lake George? I was sure Paul would go along with the idea. We never left the house in the early morning; the bathing in ice water was a big restriction. The weather was *picture perfect*, and that was a good start. Spending the day together in totally different surroundings might be good for us. I pictured a slow, relaxing walk through the village, and from there, we would see where the day led us.

I was taken away from my dream by a knock at the door. Paul entered and knelt by my bed, asked how I was, and told me he was sorry. My first instinct was to act as if I was still a little hurt, but I was quite happy with the way I felt. I told him it was okay.

From September to October 1980, I didn't bathe in any water except for my face, under my arms, and other pertinent areas.

I decided the best way to approach a fresh start was one step at a time. The thought of using any water was intimidating; however, I washed my face in tepid water, brushed my teeth, and combed my hair. I took a few deep breaths, and then I was ready to face the day. I entered the kitchen with a bounce to my step and a smile on my face. I didn't want to give Paul *too much* satisfaction after his behavior the previous day, but what I was experiencing was awesome compared to the life I had been living.

Paul continued with his cup of coffee, and we chatted while he ate breakfast. I prepared my drink and sipped it slowly, enjoying the clean, fresh taste.

Our relationship changed on that wondrous day in Lake George. The day was totally ours, with no interference from my ice ritual. We talked and laughed and walked up and down the streets. I was excited with everything I looked at; I noticed all the fine details of the buildings, the shoreline of the lake, the trees, and the people mingling about. And, most of all, we were happy. Paul was a really good friend. I was like a child with her first visit to the candy store. It was as if I'd been tied down for years, and on this day, the strings were cut. I wasn't harnessed to my bedroom for meals and taking ice baths. I was overjoyed with the fact that I was able to do anything I wanted with the day, go anywhere, and there was *no deadline for returning home*. We even took a short cruise on a huge, old-fashioned paddleboat down the Hudson River. All of this was possible because the bathing in ice water ended. Unfortunately, so had my consumption of food.

The room I turned into my *ice water bathing pit* was in bad shape. The water destroyed the furniture beyond recognition. Paul wasn't upset; he was pleased I gave up the ice. And because of my positive change, he decided to work on the furniture and spruce up the room to make it more pleasant. He wanted me to enjoy my bedroom and feel good about spending time there. Generally, veneer can't be stripped, but somehow Paul, made the entire bedroom collection look better than new — truly magnificent. He also bought me new sheets, a bedspread, and throw pillows. Then he surprised me with a new stereo system. Again and again, he said, "I want you to be happy."

I had an urge to work with a paintbrush and be somewhat creative. I completed three-paint-by-number sets, and Paul willingly framed them. This was the first time I picked up a paintbrush in over ten years. It felt wonderful to see my hand give shape to a plain white canvas and stay within the black lines. Even though it wasn't freehand, I felt a great sense of accomplishment from the project; I wanted more of the same. The room was now pretty and feminine, with lots of light.

I was excited about not using cold water to control my body heat. As long as I didn't eat and only had my lemon drink, I was fine. I attempted to stay rather calm, took long rides in the car, and only engaged in a minimal amount of walking. Doing all of this kept me in my *safe zone* and heat free. By eliminating food from my diet, I was ready for bed early and could comfortably lie down and go to sleep.

Paul was a man, and he had needs. I was a woman with needs, too, but they weren't sex. At the end of the day when I finally laid my head down to rest, the continuing desire to be cool was my only priority.

Paul had other things on his mind and probably thought I did, too. He saw a young, vibrant gal who appeared to be a flirt at times and wanted attention. She was friendly and longed for companionship. He often came to my room just as I was settling down and ready to doze off. I dreaded hearing his footsteps, fear of what would be asked of me, and wishing it would stop. It wasn't the act; it was the heat it caused. I tried to explain why I didn't want to. He said it wouldn't take a long time, thinking that would minimize the problem.

It didn't. Only a few seconds was enough for my skin to react and my head to heat up. I just knew I didn't want to use cold water again. I was trying so hard to kick my addiction. This request was very inconvenient, and for me, sex wasn't of any interest. I allowed Paul to be a part of every aspect of my life and never told him it didn't include physical intimacy.

He never insinuated I'd be asked to vacate the house, but that thought was very much a part of my decision. I always gave in, out of fear, but never enjoyed it. I so wanted his house to be my home. I wanted Paul to like me, but not intimately.

After we were together for some time, Paul told me these days come back to haunt him. He continues to feel awful about what he did. He said he would have never bothered me if he had known the induced heat I felt was so bad. In his mind, he continues to beat himself up. I don't know if he'll ever get over it. He truly didn't realize how much I was suffering, and of course, no one, not even health care professionals, could adequately explain what was happening to me.

Whenever he brings this subject up, I tell him, "I tried to rise above it all and go on with my life. It's no big deal; stuff happens. The goodness in you outweighed the small part of unpleasantness at the time. I love you now, and that's all that matters."

For over forty days, during my lemon-and-ice-water period, I had nothing but ice water with lemon and artificial sweetener.

Home aides were still coming to the house. I really didn't need them. They weren't cooking. They were no more than companions. They were supposed to make sure I ate. If Paul thought for one minute I wasn't eating, I'm sure our relationship would have exploded. He thought I was. He was at work most of the day and extremely tired when he arrived home. He assumed the aide was making sure I consumed an adequate amount of food. When we went out together, he saw that I only sipped my lemon drink.

From time to time, Paul said, "Aren't you hungry? Don't you want something to eat?"

I told him I was fine, and then I quickly changed the subject. I was deathly afraid he would attempt to make me eat. I was very happy not eating. I didn't have to worry about food making me hot, and the day was open to choice, with no confining schedule. It was a relief when he went to work. The same held true when it was time for bed.

I quietly mumbled, "Thank goodness, I got through another day without eating."

That is how scared I was. I was so afraid of eating and becoming hot; there was no way in hell I was going to eat. I'm not sure how much anyone realizes my determination. Most anyone would think a person would eventually eat. How difficult is that? I didn't give in an inch.

My home aide knew I should be eating. I pleaded with her and made her promise not to tell Paul. I told her I was fine, and I wasn't hungry. I didn't want to eat — period. She went along with me. Ultimately, he was furious she didn't tell him.

People might think a woman with motherly instincts would have insisted I eat. No one could make me eat. When I wrapped my mind around a thought, no one could change my way of thinking. If Paul had given me an ultimatum of eating or leaving his house, I would have said good-bye and been gone. The very thought petrified me, although I knew how much he cared about me, so possibly, I assumed he wouldn't let me go. In my mind, I wasn't suffering from the lack of food.

Paul and I went all over the Capital District; I had endless energy for quite some time. I was at a good weight — maybe a little overweight by my preferences. Because I was *not eating*, the weight started to fall off. I saw myself as slender, happy, pretty, alive, no addictions, and finally unbound.

Unfortunately, the addiction was still there. I just didn't know it, or I chose to ignore it. I was preoccupied with the joy of the day, not of facing my addiction to ice water and dealing with it on another level. I felt I had been through a long nightmare and finally had awakened, so why not enjoy it? I didn't want to discuss anything unpleasant; I only lived for the moment, the now.

The possibility of dying did not enter my conscious brain. Yet if a person stops eating for a long period of time, he or she will starve to death. All that mattered to me was being free of the excess heat within my body that made life close to insufferable. The lemon drink gave me sufficient energy and peace of mind; that's as far as I wanted to think.

Getting rid of the heat gave me social contacts, and it did not place restrictions on my comings and goings. I made plans, and the hour of the day didn't matter. I didn't have to worry about the after effects of eating.

I was headed toward destruction, a permanent end.

No one can live without eating; neither could I.

Almost every day, I wanted Paul to take me for a drive somewhere. This occupied the day; we were out of the house. Food wasn't an issue until Paul became hungry, and then over and over, I pacified him with an excuse that he accepted. I didn't want to stop this routine; therefore, each morning after he had his breakfast, I suggested a destination.

On one of our outings, Paul and I visited a Hudson Valley winery. It was now fall, and the weather changed into chilly, crisp, cool days. As I stepped into the winery lobby, I felt cold, but I kept quiet. Halfway through the winery tour, I felt ill. I still didn't complain. I didn't want Paul to tell me it was because I hadn't eaten any food. I was tired. My body felt heavy and difficult to move. Each step was unstable. My mind wasn't alert, and my eyes began to hurt. My head felt as if it were separated from the rest of my body, and my neck was stiff. By the end of the tour, I was chilled to the bone and couldn't get warm. I hadn't eaten for over a month.

We were sitting under a huge tent while Paul ate a small snack. He took one look at me and knew something was wrong. We immediately went to the car, and he demanded I take my body temperature. It was ninety-two degrees. I was headed for hypothermia.

I don't even remember the drive home.

I was an icicle to touch, and a hot bath wouldn't raise my body temperature. Paul's body was always warm; he radiated heat. He offered to hold me. My body temperature was so low, I desperately needed warmth, and I naturally clung to him in desperation. We lay on his bed, and I fell asleep in his loving arms. His body heat plus my condition put me to sleep. I was so warm and sleepy that I stayed there all the next day.

Paul left for work when the home aide came on duty. The only thing I remember is sleeping for days. My body was unresponsive to daylight. It was as if I had fallen into a semiconscious state. Every day was lived as if I had just gone to bed. Paul said he challenged me with questions; I didn't respond. I looked so weak. He thought it was good I rested and stayed warm, so he let me sleep.

Unfortunately, I wasn't putting in enough fuel. My body temperature was falling, and I was losing ground. When he was with me, he took my temperature periodically. I was *so out of it* that I bit down on every thermometer and broke them in half. Paul's special-order for a dozen turned out to be a wise decision; we went through enough of them.

I reached a point where I was urinating and passing stool in the bed. I had no control over my body functions. He came home from work, cleaned me up, did a load of wash, had his dinner, cleaned me up again, and did another load of wash. I vaguely remembered the hum of the washing machine as Paul moved about the room.

He was desperately worried about my nutrition, so he insisted I sit at the kitchen table while he put an assortment of foods in front of me. I refused everything. He tried tossing grapes, from a short distance, into my mouth. He said I chomped on them, pits and all.

I urinated on the kitchen chair and didn't even know it. I was unable to sign my name. Paul asked me questions, and before he finished the sentence, I was dozing off. I was at a point where I couldn't take care of myself. I wouldn't eat, and Paul had no choice but to take me back to the hospital.

Paul drove me to the emergency room and requested Dr. Howard. Luckily, she was on duty. A feeding tube was inserted, vitals taken, and I was admitted. My low body temperature always came from poor nutrition and freezing myself. This time, I was diagnosed as a hypothermia patient with anorexia nervosa.

Paul and I started to form a much stronger relationship. Paul was my best friend. He felt I needed someone to look after me, so he took on that role as well. He never missed a day of visiting me in the hospital, even though he worked all day in construction. And he made sure I always had flowers in my hospital room.

I was weighed, and my food intake was calculated daily to see if I was trying to avoid eating. As with my previous admissions, the doctors questioned why the low body temperature. Upon being admitted this time, I was 110 pounds, and my body temperature was ninety degrees. Before the absence of caloric food, I weighed 160 pounds.

Dr. Howard and several other doctors and interns were very interested in my medical case. One, in particular, wanted me to have an electroencephalogram. This was a test to view the electrical activity in the brain. I really didn't want to have it, but Paul said if they could help me in any way, I should think about agreeing to the test. It was an uncomfortable exam where they turned me upside down after inserting a needle of sorts into my spine. Once it was over, I had to lie still without moving my head for twenty-four hours. It was horrible. After the test, the pain was close to indescribable. A burning sensation ripped up my back into the neck, leaving me with a migraine that never stopped. Any turn of the head felt as if my brain were being twisted and all blood flow being blocked by a tourniquet around my neck.

I lay there with tears soaking my pillow and said to Paul, "Please, don't let me die. I think I am going to die. Please, don't let me die."

I was flat on my back for what seemed an eternity. The test established nothing but agony.

After twenty-four hours, I was encouraged to walk to the bathroom. Every step I took, I thought my head would fall off from the pain. If I didn't hold Paul's arm to steady myself, I would have fallen to the floor. Years later, I contributed my severe migraines partly to this test. I'll never be sure of it, but the possibility is real.

Then to make matters worse, I had a roommate who insisted on a warm room. Without a cool environment, I couldn't eat enough to keep a bird alive. I was miserable and continued to beg for coolness and some moving air.

One of the interns said my actions were all psychiatric. He clearly wanted me out of his ward. Paul went right after him with strong, colorful words and let him have it in detail. The intern never gave us any more problems. Unfortunately, after a battle with him and causing considerable upheaval on the unit, the nurses moved me out — bed and all. I liked the room, just not the roommate. I was upset with the decision to move me and not her. I cried and begged Paul to let me stay; after all, I was admitted first. He tried to convince me I'd be better off in a private room where I could do as I pleased with the temperature. I was afraid I couldn't eat alone, with no one else there. I had a lot of mental *baggage*; much of it was fear.

Another test was called the blanket test. The room was set at sixty-eight degrees. The technicians raised the temperature of the blanket. My body didn't respond normally; it registered 92 degrees instead of 98.6 degrees. The next phase was to lower the blanket temperature. Again, I didn't react as expected.

The hypothalamus has a variety of functions, some of which are regulating appetite, body temperature, and hormones. In anorexia nervosa patients, these three elements are mildly affected. In my case, it was more severe; so the doctors speculated I had a lesion in the hypothalamus gland, which created a very low body temperature. They were never able to establish my irregular eating habits because I didn't cooperate. When I was told to eat a specific diet for medical reasons, I never followed through. I changed my ways because of circumstances, not because someone told me to. (Sections of the case report are documented at the end of the book.)

Dr. Howard held a special conference in the small theater at the hospital. She told me she was going to describe my condition, talk about my medical history, and state her findings thus far. I would be asked to come up on stage so the audience, mostly medical personnel, could view my body. I would be asked to disrobe and show my backside, which was mostly bone, and then bend forward so the audience could view a huge area on the top of my head. The scalp showed a considerable amount of hair loss. And I had large, ugly sores throughout my scalp. I was the visual that matched the study on paper.

The nurses expected me to take sponge baths like everyone else. I was nervous about bathing. It was a symbol of my addiction, and I was afraid to begin using water on my body again. It was too easy for me to be drawn back into a daily obsession. I wouldn't consider a full bath or shower — too much water all around me. There wasn't enough time in the day to explain to the nurse my history, so I started out with a minimal amount of water and gingerly touched my body, waiting for a sign. The sponge bath was okay, but it wasn't my favorite part of the day. I was relieved a few hours later. I used to think that by then my skin was like everyone else's, normal.

My meals were monitored; the staff had to know exactly what I ate at each meal. They could not take my word for it. Dr. Howard was looking for an increase in my weight and an improvement in my blood. I was literally starving when I arrived. A nutritionally fortified diet was long overdue. I was on a feeding tube plus a regular diet. The tube feeding supplied the majority of my nutritional needs, but I was also given a tray with a hospital meal. I ate very little from the tray. I preferred the tube feedings; they didn't overheat me.

The beef flavor was extra thick, and there was always a chance of it clogging the tube. The first time it happened, we called for a nurse, and she didn't come right away. I had overheard a nurse say all the tubes need prompt attention if this happens. I was close to hyperventilating. Paul had seen the staff working with the lines many times, so without hesitation, he came over to my bedside and performed the cleaning-out procedure. I wasn't nearly as confident as he was, but he told me it was a no-choice situation. He accomplished the task perfectly. I was able to breathe easy again, and all was right with the world. He was my savior on many levels. The only time he left my side was to go to the cafeteria for something to eat.

I was given permission to go down to the cafeteria. Paul put money in the drawer next to my bed in case I decided the temptation was too great. Dr. Howard thought maybe if I tried some other foods, I would begin to eat more. She also put me on a high dosage of thiamine.

Dr. Howard's prescription of thiamine worked. I began to eat and eat and eat. The more I consumed, the warmer I became; therefore, I opened a window. And then I was able to eat more. My room became so chilly, the door leading into my room was kept closed; the other patients and nurses complained the hallway was too cold. After consuming three meals in my room, I ventured down to the cafeteria in the evening for ham and cheese sandwiches, pastries, candy bars, bread and butter, and ice cream.

I added another obsession, an evening habit. Heat took over my body after a few hours in bed. I set the alarm for one hour. When the alarm buzzed, I quickly shut if off so no one would hear it. Quietly, I tiptoed out of my room and walked up and down the halls to cool my body. As I walked, my body felt cooler. Then I returned to my bed. I set the alarm clock for another hour and walked again. I repeated this procedure all night long.

The nurses saw me walking and said, "Jill, what are you doing out of bed? You're not supposed to be walking in the halls."

I replied, "I was told I could walk anytime I wanted."

The night shift didn't like it, but I continued this obsessive behavior every night.

Days turned into weeks, and the complete hospital stay was close to three months. I became part of the woodwork. Once again, I had made my nesting place. The day had structure, which was set up by someone else and then followed by all. The liberties I was given gave me some control over my situation. I enjoyed the brief intervals of conversation with the nurses and doctors. I was always a people person, yet the addiction gave me a hermit's life. After years of torture with my own methods of survival, the hospital wasn't too bad. Of course, I thought so, too, the last time I was admitted.

I was gaining a sufficient amount of weight, and all my vital signs were good. The hospital's work was ending. Most people want to go home; I didn't. Most importantly, I was able to eat without freezing my body with cold water. And if I wanted to eat in the cafeteria, I could do that, too. I walked in the corridor — which had a very comfortable temperature setting — at any time of the day and slept when my body needed it.

Overall, I had a tremendous amount of freedom. What the hospital gave me during my stay was a gift. It was a huge part of the healing process. And I will be forever grateful to Albany Medical Center. They kept me alive physically and mentally.

I adjusted easily to the hospital's secure routine and disruption was an unhappy thought.

Home represented a struggle. I didn't listen to what my body told me. I overextended myself continuously until my body couldn't take the punishment any longer. I wasn't able to accept the temperatures, no matter where I set the thermostat. All of that had to change for the better.

For so long, I put all my faith in cold water. It got me through the day. The ice gave me life but almost took it away. And Paul felt, by removing the ice from my life, he had created a Shakespearean tragedy. I, on the other hand, felt it was a turning point in my life and a blessing in disguise. I ended up in the hospital, but I was returning to my home instead of going to the funeral parlor. I stopped surrounding myself in ice and cold water, and that was a step forward. Now, maybe, I had a chance in life.

A few days before being discharged, Paul and I were given permission to leave the hospital for the afternoon. I still had the tube feeding equipment taped to my nose. We went to a Howard Johnson's Restaurantand had brownie fudge pie with ice cream and hot coffee. This was my first time eating in a restaurant with Paul. I was quite surprised I didn't mull the thought over and weigh my alternatives. Our outing happened on the spur of the moment. If I had thought too much about it, it probably wouldn't have happened. I had chained myself to solely eating at home and wouldn't think of eating in a restaurant. It was as if I had been given a long overdue present. We were having fun together, and the food tasted marvelous. I wasn't too sure about doing it again, but that decision didn't have to be made immediately.

As Paul and I were getting ready to leave the hospital, Dr. Howard suggested I might want to consider seeing a professional for guidance, concerning some of my fears and obsessions.

I had mixed emotions about my health. At times, I thought some of my problems might be psychiatric, but there were many areas that pointed to medical. My body temperature registered eighty-eight degrees, and no one could dispute that. How warm I felt was solely my description of the heat, and people either had to take my word for it or they didn't. Paul was convinced it was medical, because I did everything imaginable just so I could eat.

To help clear up some of my thoughts, I decided to go to a psychiatrist. I didn't feel at ease with him. He sat and listened. I didn't feel any different when I left his office. I didn't see the doctor anymore, and years later I learned he committed suicide! Upon hearing that, I wondered whose issues were worse.

Paul had the patience of a cat. I put up so many barriers, but he continued to support me. He felt there was more to my condition than met the eye. Anyone watching my actions could easily diagnose me as totally *nuts*. Paul and Dr. Howard gave me the benefit of the doubt over and over again. I imagine there are many instances where a patient acts inappropriately, and immediately, they are labeled as such. The underlying issues are often missed or not even asked about. A patient's vital signs are monitored. What is seen by the naked eye is acted upon. This is all standard procedure. To look into the more complicated reason of why he or she is acting abnormally may sometimes be overlooked. I found that what is happening *right now* is the only thing some physicians are interested in. Thank God, my doctor was different.

Chapter 14
Back Home Again

I was still on the feeding tube when I left the hospital. A supply of canned food, along with instructions, accompanied me home. I wasn't to be trusted eating adequately on my own.

The nutritional supplement had to move through the plastic line and end up in my stomach. It wasn't a fast process. Sitting and doing nothing wasn't one of my best qualities. I didn't knit in years, but now it seemed a good time to start. Paul was delighted to see me interested in a project that involved sitting instead of moving. Whatever was needed for my progress, Paul tried to accommodate me. He suggested a shopping spree the next day for yarn and more needles.

The feedings didn't taste as good as they did in the hospital, and I lost my appetite. Paul didn't think I was consuming a sufficient amount of food, so he frequently asked what I was eating. The constant monitoring of my consumption became annoying. I felt I was eating enough, and I grew tired of food being the main conversation. All my life, I had trouble keeping my weight where I wanted it to be; I was always careful of what I ate. I never saw myself as too thin.

It was nice to occasionally eat an item I might not ordinarily eat. But that didn't mean I was going to do it all the time. I was continuously encouraged to eat and, for all the right reasons, to stay alive. At this point in time, I could afford to eat weight-gaining foods and not feel guilty about putting on a few extra pounds. That is what I said, but it wasn't necessarily what I really believed. I didn't want to see the scale read too high by my standards. I never wanted to be heavy again. A little weight was okay, but not too much. Plus I still had the *heat* problem, which dictated the foods I could tolerate.

The term *anorexia nervosa* didn't sit well with Paul.

He questioned me as to whether I thought I was, and I'd always retaliate with "No, I am not anorexic. I want to eat; I just get too hot."

The topic subsided for a while. But it didn't disappear. I knew how he felt. I almost feared how he felt. It was really important to Paul that I eat and stay out of the hospital. He said it was as simple as that. I knew if I didn't eat and ended up back in the hospital, I might lose him.

I put these past sentences in for a reason. If anyone reads between the lines, there are definitely anorexic tendencies. What I previously wrote was exactly what I was thinking at the time. No one could convince me I was anorexic. Another doctor working with Dr. Howard said I did have eating issues along with other conditions. We couldn't completely dismiss the possibility of anorexia nervosa. He was examining the whole picture of my medical condition. Addressing the low body temperature was extremely important. I needed to be aware of the danger involved when I didn't eat an adequate amount of food or allowed myself to become too cold. All I heard was the word "anorexia," and I became very upset.

My next question, "Why does it have to be anorexia? Isn't there something else that pertains to me?"

I heard only what I wanted to hear. I didn't want to be categorized with an unhealthy label. The doctor told me the word "anorexia" was bothering me more than seeing where I was in my life at the moment. The past was gone. We were working on the *now* and my future. If I let myself deteriorate again and allow my nutrition to suffer and the body temperature to drop, I could put myself right in the category of a name I didn't like. I had eating issues, which placed me with anorexia patients.

Finally, the doctor got the message across, and I seemed to understand, and I was okay with it as long as we both agreed I wasn't anorexic.

I stated *both* for a particular reason: anorexia patients are known to be controllers. I was controlling the doctor's thinking along with mine. I felt at peace as long as I knew he felt the same way I did. Even though he might not have, in my mind that is what I was thinking. If I said *both*, then I knew we were *both* on the same page.

My thinking on this matter was from an *addict's* point of view, and I was in denial. Try to express a rationale to a person who lives with an obsession. The person who is trying to help slides into the position of a therapist. A friend, or therapist, goes over the reasoning again and again and again. The helper thinks his or her point has been made and is agreed upon because the obsessed individual nods during the entire conversation. When the discussion is over, the person with the obsession makes a remark that shows he or she hasn't changed his or her thinking at all. The patient is steadfast to what he or she says no matter what anyone else says.

Everything I proclaimed seemed totally logical and medical to me, versus psychiatric. Survival was obviously normal, as far as I was concerned. At times, I felt as if I were on the witness stand defending myself. I went head-to-head with anyone who questioned what I believed to be true. I was a very stubborn lady.

Slowly, as I came to terms about my past, I realized maybe I did lean toward the condition of anorexia nervosa. I never wanted to see myself overweight — never mind what the scale said. At times, I talked as if I ate a banquet when it was merely enough to keep a bug alive.

The question of what foods to consume so I could still function, was an ongoing dilemma. I often blamed food for a good day or bad day. When I overate, I thought it showed immediately. I made an attempt to take off the newly gained weight as quickly as possible. When I ate a dessert, I felt guilty. Then I punished myself by eating twice as much as I needed, and then continued to binge.

My troubled mind thought, "Now that I've eaten what I shouldn't, I might as well keep on going and have a grand ol' time. I've screwed up my diet anyway. " As if gorging myself beyond sensibility was logical.

Sometimes I'm amazed at how my brain rationalized situations. There were definitely eating issues in my life; however, I went through a lot of suffering just so I could eat. I don't know Dr. Howard's exact assessment of my case, but lucky for me, she was in my corner. I know that as her patient, I was very strong-willed in my deep-rooted thinking and would put up barriers as soon as she tried to help, even when I was faced with the truth.

I've never met any doctor like her. She is truly a magnificent, caring, compassionate, and highly educated doctor.

Tests and observation indicated there was a possibility of a lesion in the brain, which could have caused the temperature imbalance. Or I could have caused such problems using cold water. But nothing explained why I felt hot when my body thermometer read normal or below normal. Exploratory surgery to investigate the lesion was risky, and there was no way to guarantee it would offer a cure for my problems. I did not pursue any surgery inside my head, and we never knew exactly what happened or in what order.

Paul prepared the evening meal. The home aide was with me for lunch. The supplemental feedings continued. Before long, they filled my stomach up too much, and I didn't want to eat anything else. On top of everything else, I was having frequent headaches.

One night, I started to vomit. It was't a good thing to have food come back up through the tube. I was petrified, and I didn't know what to do. I knew the tube line was clogging with vomit. A doctor should have been there to remove it, but there wasn't enough time. It had to be done right then and there.

I called Paul, and once again, he took care of the situation. I was worried and frightened, but he had complete confidence and managed it beautifully. If the tube lines aren't handled correctly, they can do severe damage to the lung. In time of need, Paul was there as usual. He stepped forward and, without hesitation, corrected the problem.

I was falling for this man. He was just plain terrific. When I relayed to Dr. Howard what Paul did, she was impressed. Then the doctor added, Paul was often 50 percent right and 50 percent wrong, and sometimes she wished she had listened to him.

The tube feedings ended that day. Paul left a pot of bouillon on the stove, hoping I would indulge frequently. He encouraged me to drink as much as possible so my body temperature would stay up. I drank much more than my body could handle, and the high salt content made my ankles swell up like balloons. I refused to take a hot bath, and Paul prayed the hot liquids would suffice. The objective was to keep the body temp normal.

Each time I sat down for dinner, the kitchen appeared to be shrinking. The closed in feeling created more heat than I could cope with. I yearned for cold air or cold water. I didn't want to give in to the latter. For now, I was managing a light breakfast and lunch without cold water. I told Paul I couldn't eat our big meal at home anymore. It wasn't working. I thought it was time for a drastic change.

We went *down river* to visit my father. On our way home, I saw a familiar restaurant — one I had gone to many times over the years. I suggested we stop and have dinner. Paul was delightfully surprised. I wanted to shout, "I'm eating out in a restaurant."

We had steak, potatoes, vegetables, and salad for dinner. Paul ordered a beer, and I thought, why not? So I had one, too. We had coffee and cheesecake for dessert. I was thrilled; I ate a whole meal in a restaurant without cold water. Cool air moved about the room, which helped a great deal.

The restaurant experience was an eye opener. It led to many more similar evenings all around the Capital District. Each time we dined out, I saw that my food consumption was improving, and so began our restaurant tour. It had been years since I had eaten a full-course meal in a restaurant. The last time was around 1970, as I remembered, so this was a huge advancement in my healing.

I was fixated with eating out, and I refused to eat at home. I just couldn't bring myself to do it. My appetite was much better, and I was gaining a considerable amount of weight. We dined all over the Capital District from steak houses to seafood restaurants, and from fine dining to quick and fun places.

After sampling many eateries, we generally concentrated on the favorite — the one with the coolest air temperature. When a restaurant didn't produce enough circulating air, I devised an alternative plan. I decided to walk outdoors in the cool air before going in.

The air was cool for sure, and it was soothing as long as I was outdoors; however, the exercise was creating internal heat. As with any workout, heat builds up. When you stop, you feel hot. That is what happened to me. As I walked outdoors, I obtained the coolness I needed; but when I entered the building, I was overheated.

After Paul and I were seated, I waited to cool off; then I burped and felt cooler. I assumed the burp was a sign of cooling off. Therefore, in my mind, I came to the conclusion I had to do that every time we went out to eat. Sometimes, I didn't burp. Excusing myself from the table, I meandered into the bathroom in hopes of a result. If it didn't happen, I pounded my stomach until I burped. Sometimes, I couldn't burp at all but continued to pound my stomach.

Then my face flushed, and I became uncomfortably hot. I was so upset, the food didn't taste good, and I ate very little. During each excursion to the restroom, I was absent from the table for quite a long time. Upon returning, Paul always asked what was wrong. I was embarrassed to tell him, so I said I was fine; I really wasn't fine at all.

I had incorporated a new obsession, and I didn't even know it. This went on for some time. It didn't stop until I was sick at home for several days. The next time we returned to a restaurant, I didn't feel like walking outdoors first. The need to burp finally stopped, too. In the past, Paul told me many times the walking was giving me a terrible temperature change. I didn't listen.

Swimming in cold water had ruled my very existence for many years; it allowed me to eat. I no longer had it as an insurance policy. If, by chance, an incident occurred where my body remained cool, I hung on to the event, and then it was incorporated into an obsession. As I worked at stopping one obsession, I usually incorporated another one.

I don't ever remember changing because someone suggested it. All my changes normally came from unpleasant situations where I was forced to alter my daily routine.

We even went dancing several times. Normally, I was up on the floor for every dance. Even though I became warm from the dance moves, I felt cooler when I was moving. One night, my ankles were so swollen from Paul's pot of bouillon that I had to sit out all the dances. Paul got up and danced alone, to a very groovy tune, all around my table. It didn't bother him in the least, dancing alone. He loved it, and the crowd in the club seemed to enjoy his freedom of expression, although his spontaneity was a little difficult for me to get used to at times. I had never been around such a free spirit. Maybe this trait enabled me to be more at ease with him than any other male.

These date nights, together with the dancing, were also very romantic.

Over time, eating in restaurants lost its sparkle. My days consisted mostly of waiting for dinner so I could be out of the house and moving around. I felt as if I wanted to get away from myself; however, the heat always followed me everywhere. Eat, walk, eat, walk, and then finally go to bed. There was nothing else to look forward to in the day.

We were together all the time, and we ran out of conversation. Paul didn't like gaining weight. It cost a lot of extra money to eat out regularly, especially at the times when he was laid off from work. He decided to eat at home to save money and then join me while I ate out.

Dining out actually became another obsession or maybe even an addiction, and I wasn't able to stop. Now I believed I had to eat out. Paul suggested eating at home many times. My mind was made up even before he finished his sentence. I would not discuss the possibility. It had taken me years to eat enough food to be healthy without using cold water, so whatever the procedure was, at any given time, I was determined to continue in my own way — period, end of statement. The problem was I no longer enjoyed a meal unless I had a glass of wine or a beer to induce my appetite. In the past, a small amount of alcohol always increased my appetite, and a binge would follow. Now wasn't any different. The food consumption was out of control. My weight was no different. At the end of the day, I couldn't stop eating. It was as if an addictive chemical was in the food; I had to eat more and more.

Late at night, when the house was quiet, and I was alone, I had cravings for something sweet. I couldn't eat a meal at home, but I could snack. I never snacked when someone else was in the kitchen, only when I was alone.

I took a little ice cream, and before I knew it, a whole quart was gone. That wasn't satisfying, so I ate a candy bar and more ice cream. I switched to a sandwich and then back to sweets. A similar pattern was seen in the past. I tried to hide what I was doing; I was ashamed I didn't have control over my eating habits. Once this scenario began, it was like a freight train without brakes. A crash was near.

The next day, when I told Paul all about it, he said, "Oh, Bengie was with you last night." Whenever I complained of overeating, he had the same comment. "Oh, Bengie's back."

I wasn't too happy with myself; however, he did lighten the mood. I couldn't help but chuckle at the way he said it.

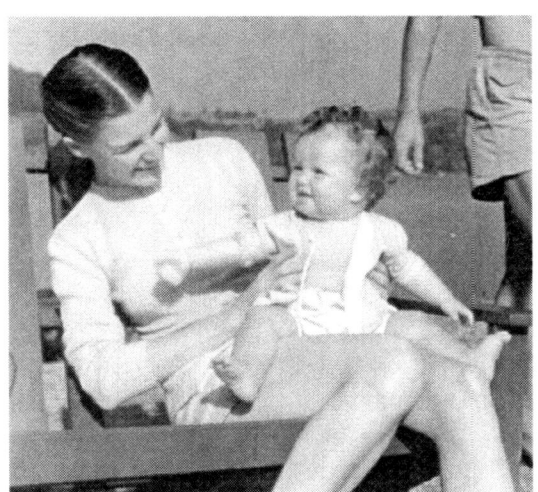

Mom and Me – Copake Lake, NY 1947

My favorite place on the planet!

Mom and Me – Copake Lake, NY 1949

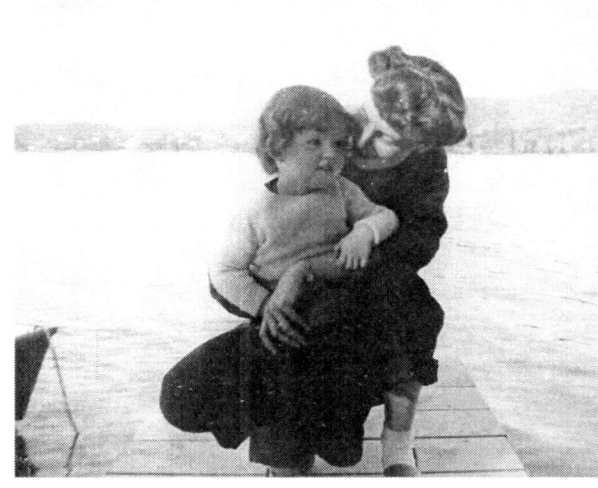

Dad and Me – Father/Daughter Weekend, Endicott Jr. College 1967

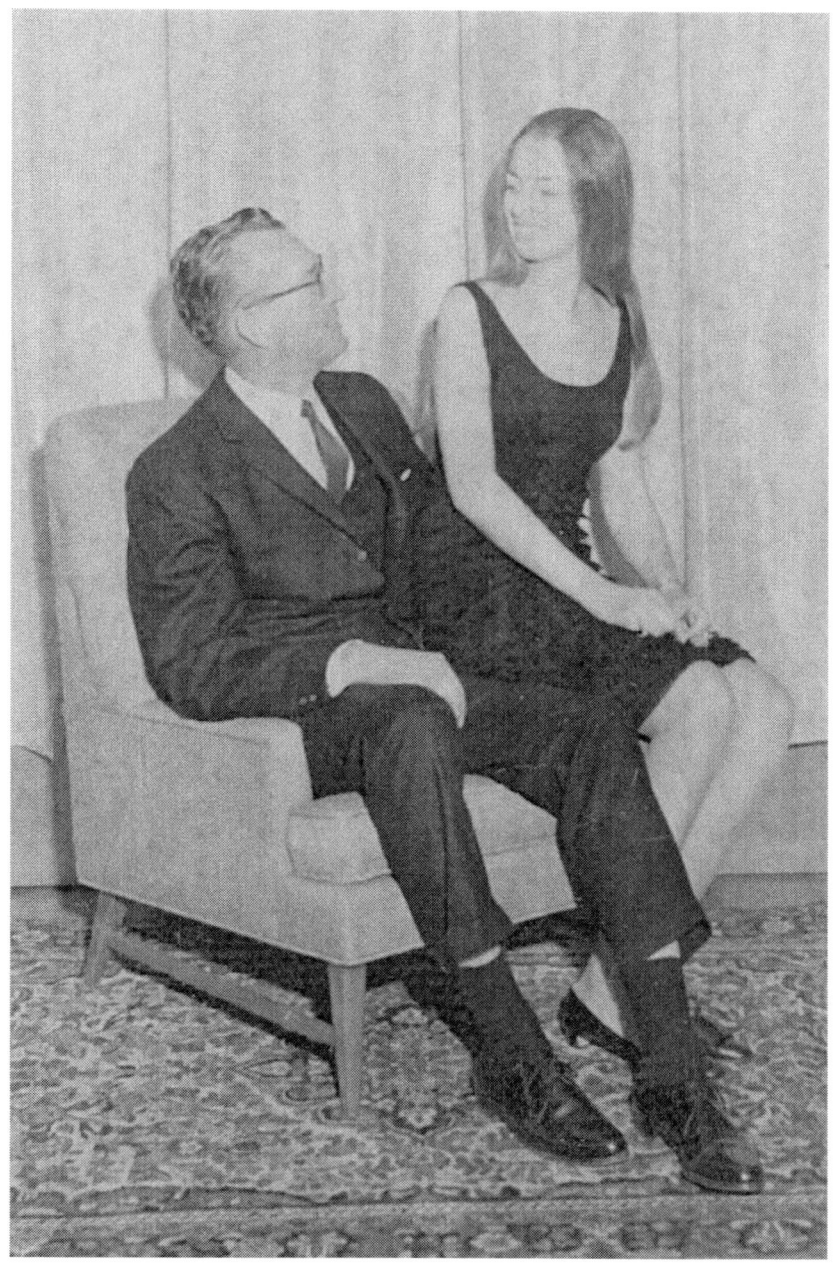

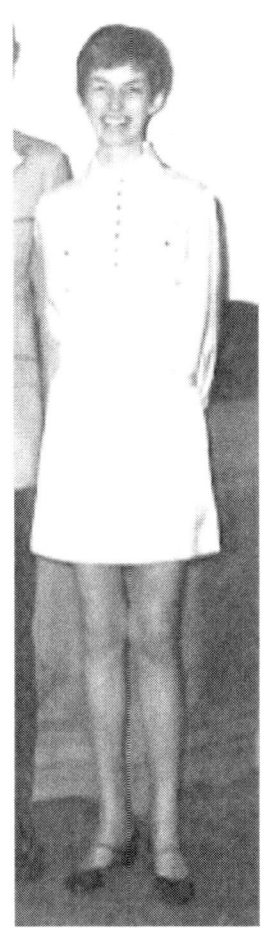

After my return from New York City, 1968 – 110 pounds

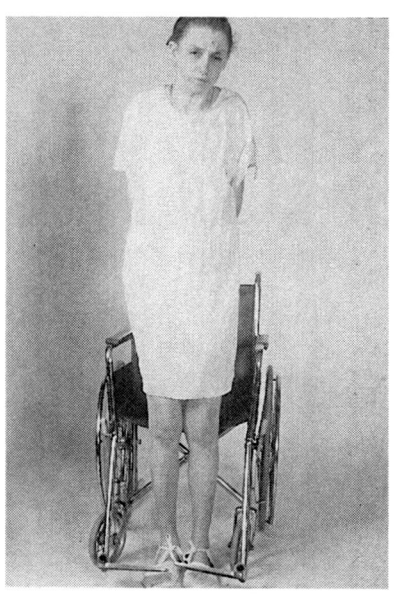

Me at medical conference at Albany medical Center, Albany, New York
January 19, 1980

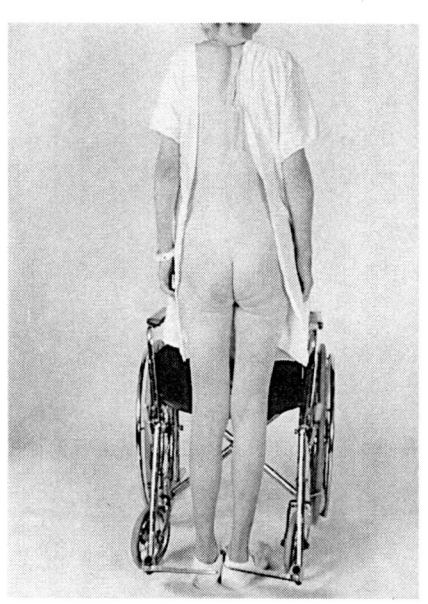

My new friend and
angel on earth, Paul, 1980

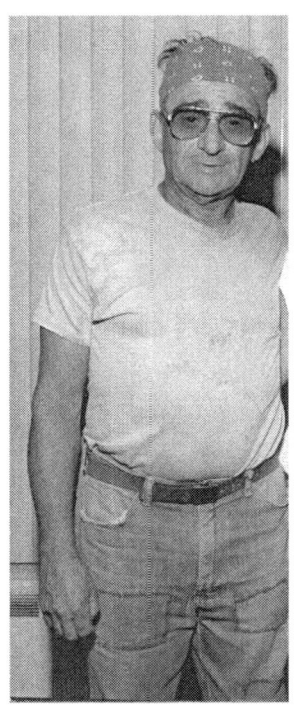

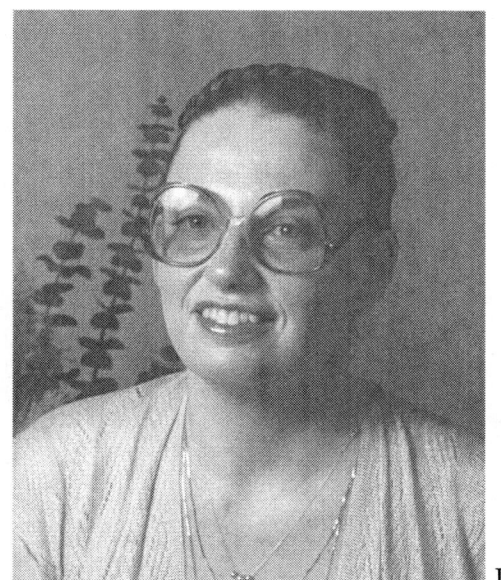

I weighted 190 pounds. Someone asked if I was pregnant, so I went on my own severe weight loss program. 1980

Paul and Jill on their wedding day
March 25, 1988

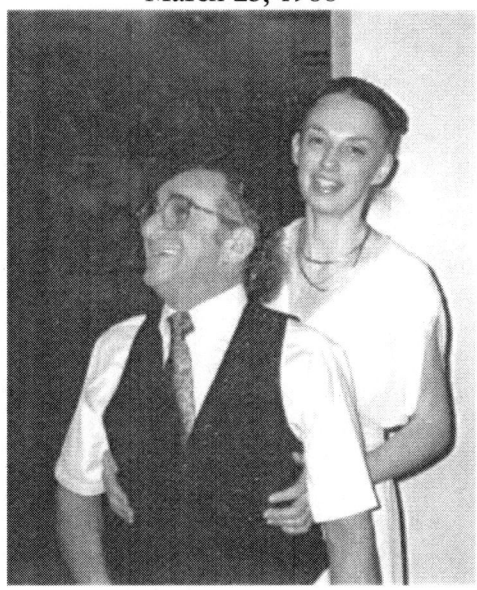

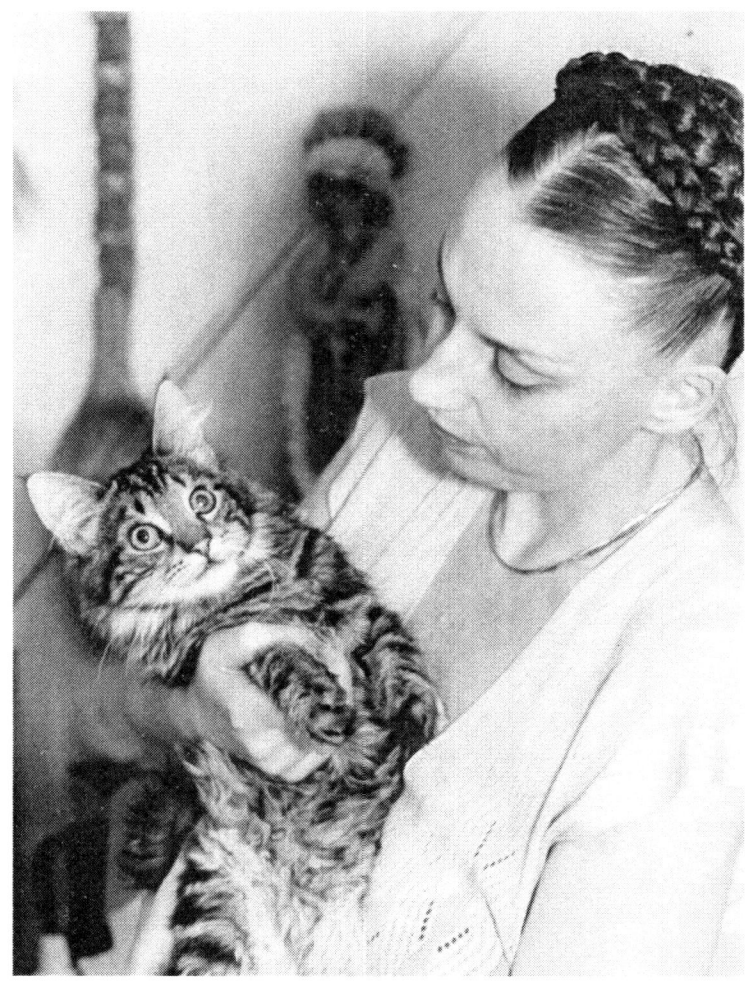

Pepper, our Maine Coon cat and me.
August 1985

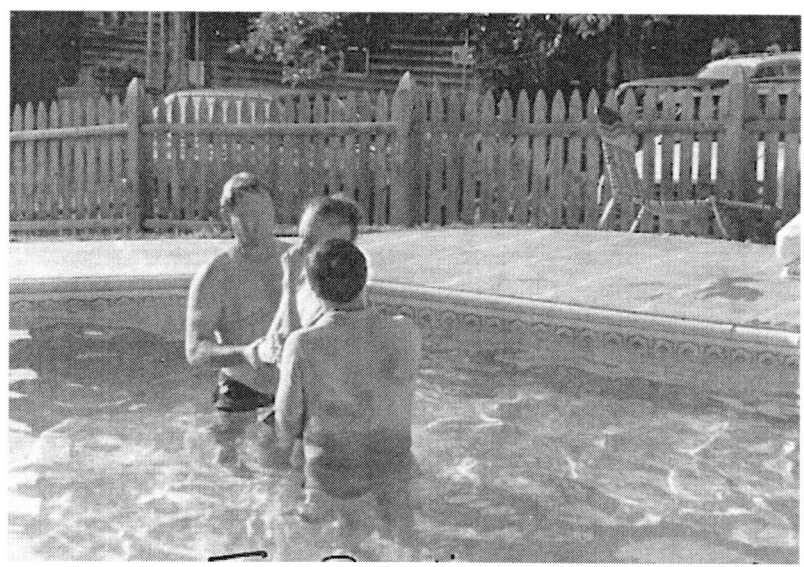

Water Baptism – July, 1988

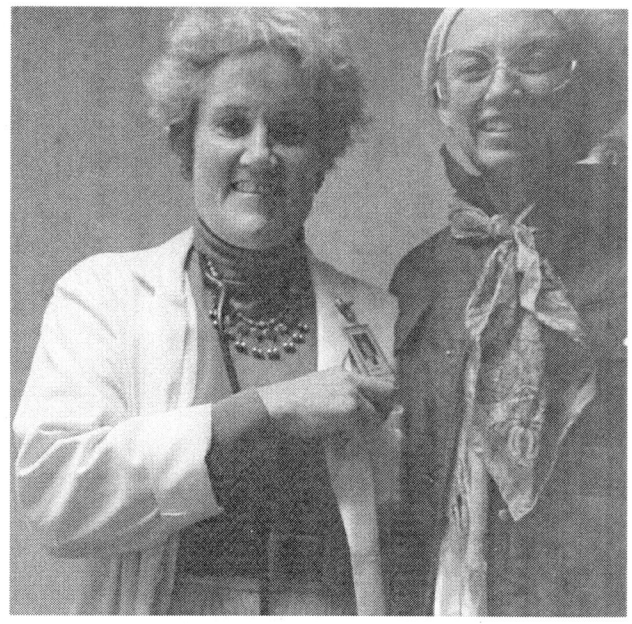

Dr. Howard and Jill - 1994

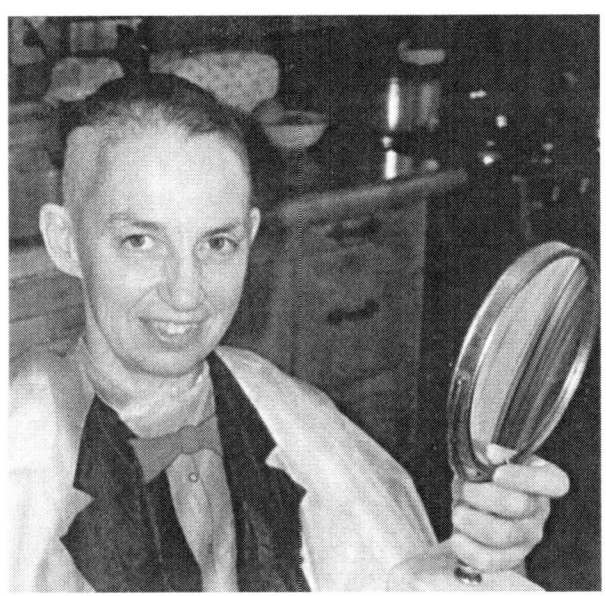

After a haircut by Paul, 1996

Painted every room in the house with the hat on, 1997-98

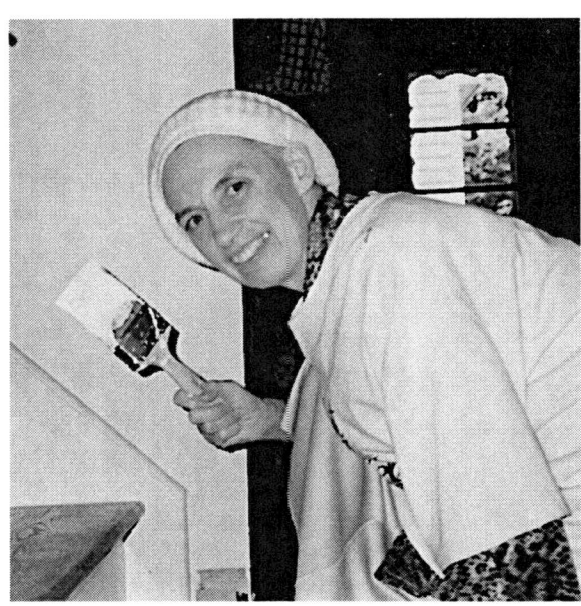

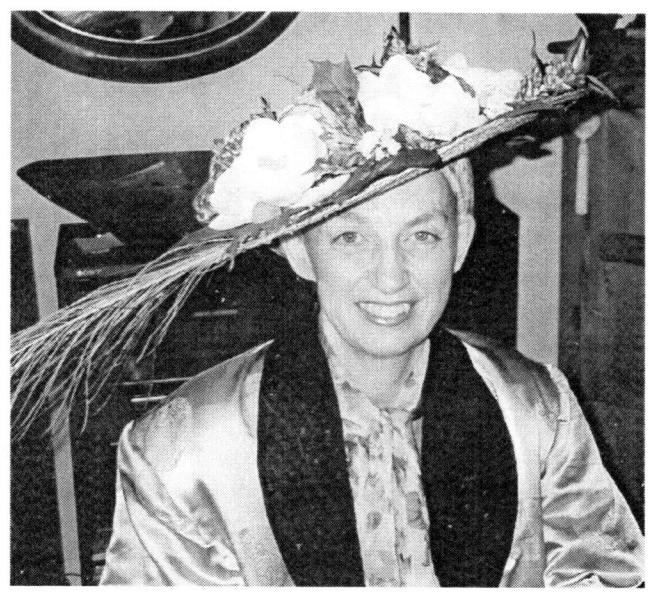

I decorated a hat for Dr. Howard's wedding, 1995
(the white hat is being hidden by a scarf under the hat)

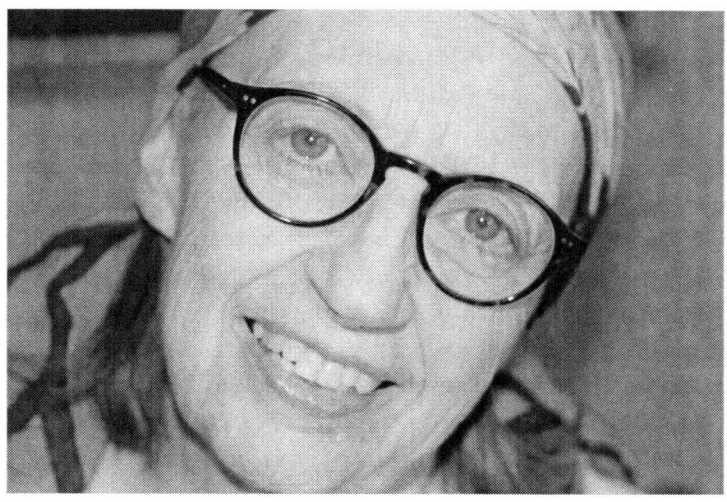

Self-portrait, Summer, 2011

Chapter 15
Hot and Heavy

Paul and I were invited to a family gathering in the summer of 1981. I overheard one of the guests ask if I was expecting. The remark hurt my feelings. I was devastated that people thought I looked fat enough to be carrying a child. At that point, any goodness I felt about myself withered away. I took a good look in the mirror; I knew I was getting too heavy at 190 pounds, and this remark confirmed it.

A had great faith in a previous diet, the one in New York City. It produced excellent results when I worked in New York City, so why not now?

I wasn't sure I still had a copy in my possession, but I found it in storage from one of our trips *down river*. It was ironic one of my belongings happened to be a copy of the diet.

Richard Simmons was popular with his exercise to music. I was determined to lose some weight. Every night, I was very diligent in practicing his entire routine. His enthusiasm was contagious. I believed in everything he said and it paid off. Maybe my serotonin levels increased, because my mood, appetite and sleep improved. I hadn't moved my body this way in years, and I was amazed how much healthier I felt by doing his workout.

I was probably more unyielding with what I ate than anyone you will ever meet. I didn't detour off my diet one iota. I was extremely careful every day and followed the diet explicitly. I didn't cheat or eat anything that wasn't on the diet, especially an item that *might* make me warm. My diet wasn't a fad or a temporary weight loss plan; it became a lifestyle *every day* for years. That is how afraid I was of becoming too warm *and* gaining all the weight back.

The view was changing. It was positive and refreshing for once in my life. The new *me* was taking a much different profile, and I felt very good about it. I had a lot more energy and was able to think with clarity. It was nice to be focused on something other than watching my body temperature and dealing with hot. As luck would have it, the exercise made me very warm; but I learned to accept it, knowing a sugar-free drink followed.

The absence of sugar in the drink was great for cooling down. I had to be careful in the wintertime because the cold liquid without any calories chilled my body to the point of lowering my body temperature. Once I realized this, I added more layers of clothing and made sure the house was warm.

The only problem was I became attached to a specific garment: a green, zippered sweatshirt. This type of clothing wasn't usually part of my wardrobe because of the type of material. It tended to create too much heat. This one didn't affect me that way, and I felt I was wearing a piece of clothing like other people. I had good days when I wore this garment; consequently, I wore it even when it was thin and full of holes. Buying new was always a challenge. The uncertainty created some fear. Other than being fanatical about one such garment, I felt this particular time in my life was finally a healthy one. Paul agreed.

When I first came to live with Paul, I didn't want anyone to see or talk to me in the morning. I needed a straight shot to cold. Then I immediately ate my breakfast. Now I was at a place in my life where the urgency wasn't as strong. Because of this, I was able to spend more time with Paul before he left for work.

This small step was another move toward my goal of becoming ordinary. I didn't have a compulsive need *at the crack of dawn* to do my thing involving water. I was able to relax and talk, while Paul drank his coffee. I also prepared a special lunch for him and included a friendly note with a smiley face. I wanted him to think of me and know how much I cared.

From 1981 to 1988, I took a hot bath
followed by three cool to cold sponge baths once a day.

I also decided it was time to take a hot bath and eliminate the warm sponge baths. When I made the attempt to bring something new into my life, it was done on my *alone* time. Not sure why, probably due to my insecurity. If the change was my idea, my confidence increased when I was the only one in the room and had no interruptions until it was complete. The first bath began one morning after Paul left for work. I thought about it, prior to his leaving, and was rather excited at the possibility. I watched his car until it disappeared from sight. Then I read or watched a soap opera to quiet myself and intensify the anticipation. Very slowly, I approached the bathroom and stared at the tub. Thoughts entered my mind as to the decision. Is today the right time for this? Am I ready? I finally took a hot bath. It did feel wonderful, at least, until I stepped out of the tub. The hot water was still on my skin. As I towel dried my body, the heat remained. Leaving the bathroom, I moved slowly to the bedroom. Now what? I had to rid myself of the heat. I could never eat a meal feeling this much heat. I knew not to panic. I was alone and had plenty of time to figure this out. And I was wiser. There had to be a way to cool down.

I slipped back into my nightgown. In order to cool off, I lay down on the bed. After about ten minutes, I slowly went down the stairs.

I sat at the kitchen table for about five minutes. Departing from the upper level to the main floor created a temperature change that warmed me up. Sitting allowed my body to adjust.

I left the kitchen and went down five steps to the lower level of the house where there was a deep sink in the laundry room. Behind closed doors, I took a sponge bath in cool water. The cool water felt too good — a tease from the past. I was sure a little cool water was okay. I wouldn't let it get out of hand.

Back upstairs in the kitchen, I sat at the table for a few minutes. I didn't feel quite cool enough.

I returned to the deep sink. Once again, I took a sponge bath in cold water.

When I finished, I returned to the kitchen and sat for a few minutes. I felt a little too warm to eat. I had to make one more trip. No one was watching. What would it hurt to ad one more trip? Back down to the deep sink for another sponge bath, again in very cold water. Once finished, I was satisfied with the ritual. At this point, I decided it was mandatory; every morning, three trips to the sink for a cold water sponge bath.

At each bathing session, I made sure I went over my entire body with a cold, wet washcloth three times — on some warm days, up to five times.

The number of times was extremely important. Three was the magical number for the cooling process.

I knew I was going too far with the obsession, but I could not cut back.

After completing all the bathing, I quickly ate my breakfast. All the food was prepared prior to the bathing. The less I exerted myself, the better it was for staying cool. If anything detained me or heated me up along the way, I had to start the process all over.

Most anyone would probably think this was an awful ordeal to go through. I was happy to have found a way to eat. I looked forward to this routine on most days; once it was over, I had a beautiful, bountiful breakfast full of healthy satisfying foods.

This was the breakfast routine 365 days a year for seven years.

When I developed a severe migraine, the obsessive-compulsive water ritual stopped. It was actually a nice break for one day. The only thing I consumed was bouillon and Coke. Without the bathing, I was afraid to eat anything of substance — again, the fear of heat.

The routine after breakfast was also consistent. Each chore was performed in the same order each day. Even though we weren't married, my household responsibilities were increasing. I was gaining self-confidence as I took on more responsibilities each day. I was cooking, cleaning, caring for our cat, and whatever else I thought I could tackle. I wanted to show Paul, and myself, that I was improving.

The cats name was Keefer. We acquired him on one of the trips *down river*. He was living with my parents. Keefer was a beautiful, golden, Maine Coon with a perfect personality. He had been an indoor cat, who occasionally slipped out the door by mistake. Paul decided he was going to train Keefer to stay on our property. Paul only worked with him for a couple of days. He never left our lot, and he always came when we called him. Keefer loved to smell the grass and lay in the sunshine while a gentle breeze ruffled his fur. I always thought he made a perfect picture.

Keefer changed our lives, and we fell in love with him. We were now a family of three. He enjoyed being near us, and the feeling was mutual. In the evening, Paul and I sat at the kitchen table, watching television. Keefer always landed in Paul's lap and fell asleep there. He had a personality that drew everyone in. He was the best of the best, and everybody adored him.

When it was time for bed, Paul said to Keefer, "Time to go night-night."

Keefer went straight to Paul's bed. He curled up at the bottom, waiting for Paul to get under the covers. Paul lifted up the sheets, creating a tent affect, and Keefer scooted under and headed for the area next to Paul's feet. Keefer's soft fur was always comforting.

One summer, Paul was working in Albany, where he was the foreman on a government project. He had a good hardworking crew. At the end of the day, they all gathered in the alley with their musical instruments for a jam session. They always had a few beers or wine, and one time, when Paul arrived home, he was feeling pretty good. I was cooking Cornish game hens for dinner. I had to leave the house early for a doctor's appointment. I left a note on the table, asking Paul to baste the hens from time to time. Then make sure the oven was off when the timer buzzed. He and Keefer were in charge. When I came home, I found an empty wine bottle on the table, and the two of them were out like a light on Paul's bed. It didn't take too much figuring to come to a conclusion. I thought they both got into the bottle of wine! The hens were the best ones we ever had, and I don't know how that happened.

The home aides continued to come five days a week. Generally, they arrived before breakfast. They were now part of my daily pattern. I depended on their companionship, but I didn't really need them. For many years, I insisted on eating alone; I didn't want people watching my unorthodox routine. In the hospital, it was the opposite. I became used to people. Those days went well, so I insisted on the same at home.

Unfortunately, I had picked up yet another new obsession. I convinced myself I couldn't go through the morning routine of bathing three times in cool water before eating my breakfast unless someone was sitting at the kitchen table. When home aide cancelled or didn't show up, I panicked. Immediately, I went to Paul for help, and I assumed he would fix the problem. I expected him to find a substitute no matter what it took. My heart rate increased, my hands perspired, I was warmer than usual, and I wouldn't eat until someone was with me. The person couldn't be elsewhere in the house. He or she had to be seated at the table. When Paul was working, he often hired a neighbor to come over and sit at the table.

Of course, most people thought I was crazy; there had to be something desperately wrong with me. For me, it wasn't mental; it was physical. On weekends, and when he wasn't working, poor Paul sat at the table and waited patiently for me to go through this obsessive behavior. He always gave up what he might want out of the day so my daily obsessions went as well as possible.

After eating breakfast, doing the breakfast dishes, making the bed, and putting the house in order, I once again lay straight out on my bed for a few minutes to cool. Then I was ready to get dressed and face the world.

Chapter 16
Fast Food Landing Pad

Each day was planned out. I felt safe by putting all parts of the day in a neat agenda. All restaurants serve coffee. Coffee has no calories. Caffeine creates energy. I enjoyed the taste. Good choice. A fast food restaurant was a nice place to sit and sip leisurely. I was part of the public buzz. It felt good. Then I was off to a nearby mall with lots of space — great for exercise and window-shopping. I was blessed with long legs. I enjoyed extended strides and feeling the air rush past my body — a pleasant experience that richly enhanced the day.

After seeing the same faces day after day, I had many new friends from the mall. Our conversations were brief but worthwhile. I chatted non-stop when Paul came home from work. My eventful day was worth sharing as far as I was concerned. I'm not so sure he felt the same; however, he always gave me time to speak my voice. He was only employed when union hall had a job for him; therefore, full-time work was sporadic. When Paul wasn't working, he tagged along with me. We were like Mutt and Jeff — such a difference in height and build.

I continued to eat in restaurants — fast food restaurants. My new diet didn't include their food so I packed my prepared dinner in a canvas bag. I wanted to be centralized and not run all over the Capital Region. Price was a factor, and I needed a place where bringing in my own food was less conspicuous. The room temperature was most important. After visiting a few, I chose a well-known chain that was close to the house. I guess I was rather obvious in the *odd* category of human beings. People whispered and stared. It wasn't on my mind that I'd be so noticeable. I was preoccupied with my accomplishments, and eating a healthy dinner. Both took priority over what people thought.

I was slowly tolerating the excess heat caused by exertion. Instead of dwelling on the heat, I created a method to lessen it. After I packed my bag, I went to the coolest room in the house and stretched out on a bed for about fifteen minutes. That was enough time to cool my body down. I headed out around four o'clock. I became such a faithful customer that I called the manager, and some of the help, by his or her first name. I arrived at the *same* time daily; sat at the *same* table; and ordered the *same* thing, which was a diet soda, a light beer, and a hot beverage. These beverages completed my healthy dinner. I didn't see anything wrong with bringing my own food as long as I ordered something. The manager didn't mind. The customers were sometimes unkind.

The fact that I ordered a beer was rather odd. Beer adds calories, and it's a carbohydrate, which creates heat, but I had an explanation for everything I did! I only drank half of a light beer. This was acceptable on my weight reduction program, and it eliminated feeling guilty about my indulgence. The restaurant temperature needed to be very cold; otherwise, drinking beer in a warm room gave me a headache and created too much heat in my body. A few sips of beer whetted my appetite so I ate a sufficient amount — but too much increased my appetite, and I ate more than I wanted to. While I was drinking the beer, I felt cool. The carbohydrates created excess warmth in my body, so I finished my meal with a considerable amount of cantaloupe, strawberries, and an apple. This lessened the heat. I was always aware of *cause and effect.*

My biggest meal of the day was at four o'clock. If I thought for one minute I had to eat that much food in my own home, it never would have happened. I was determined not to use any cold water other than the morning ritual. If this meant eating in a restaurant, then that is what would occur for as long as necessary.

Paul often told me to put the house temperature wherever I wanted it. I still had a phobia about eating at home. I couldn't bring myself to sit at the table and eat in my own home. I didn't have the answer to his "Why not?" Something different happened when I sat in a restaurant. No matter how ridiculous it sounded, I wanted to hold on to the feeling and progress from here. I felt secure knowing that what I needed would be there the next day and the day after that. I could count on it. This is what I told myself anyway.

I had more time to enjoy the simple pleasures of the day, even if it was doing nothing but to take in the view. So many years had passed where this was non-existent. I was consumed by an obsession that blocked out life. Now, I was able to take myself out of my head for a while and fit in with society.

Unfortunately, when you least expect it, your perfect moment can be whisked away. This happened from time to time when silly teenagers thought it was smart to make fun of me. I brought my own food into a restaurant. The clothes I wore were similar each day. The hairstyle I chose was a bit different than most. When I observed the snickering and giggles, the long stares, and occasionally read lips, it was easy to assess what they were saying. I guess I made their day. At first, they took me off guard. They hurt my feelings and spoiled the joyful mood I was in. But after awhile, I ignored their stupidity and adolescence.

What mattered most? I was more than okay with my progress. I felt safe and loved. Paul and Keefer were my world, and with both of them at my side, I was going to succeed. Each time I drove down Forts Ferry Road, I looked forward to pulling into our driveway. Keefer's cute, little face was usually in the living room window. He was waiting for Mommy's hug and some dinner.

I believe I stood taller as the months moved along. There was confidence in each step I took. My body was welcoming the change.

Slowly but surely, the house became my haven. Paul let me rearrange the furniture and redecorate within our meager budget. I was actually living with a man in his house. The meaning of words didn't seem real or easy to accept as true. And yet, there it was right in front of me — rather awesome. Paul's house was our home.

My habitual routine outside the house took up a considerable amount of time. Paul probably would have enjoyed me being at home more, but he accepted my lifestyle.

During this period, Paul and I had a wonderful relationship. My fondness for him grew, as our lives became genuinely intertwined.

I am twenty years younger, yet I never thought of him as being older. He was amazing: alert, active, endless energy, sharp mind, and not afraid to tackle any project. He had more get-up-and-go than I did.

Paul gave so much of himself. His patience, relentless unselfishness, care, and unconditional love were always present. He played an enormous role in my growth of becoming an independent woman. After I filed bankruptcy, it wasn't long before he applied for a credit card on his account. I received a card in my name. This was a big part of the process towards my independence, if I wanted it. I couldn't have asked for a better man and friend.

Paul belonged to the laborers' union, and work was sporadic. Whenever the telephone rang, Paul said it meant money, and a laborer was glad to take anything that was offered. Paul tried to be with me all the time or saw to it that someone was. He said I was number one, and my needs came first. He even turned down jobs when no sitter was available. My fluctuating body temperature scared him; it dropped too easily, and it was even more difficult to bring back up; therefore, he didn't want me to be left alone.

Paul and I were falling in love. It was as simple as that. He told me that he loved me first.

He said, "I fell in love with you the first day I met you. Standing in my kitchen, you looked so thin and frail. You were wearing the polka-dotted sundress you loved so much; a pair of well-worn, well-traveled sandals; and an old, thin raincoat. The vision of that day will always be in my thoughts. Even before you said much, I knew I liked you a lot."

On one of our return trips from *down river*, a strong desire came over me. I couldn't stop it; neither did I want to stop it. Every day, I was attracted to him more and more, and the longing was getting the best of me. I hadn't felt a need for sexual satisfaction since my first days of swimming in cold water. Now, those urges were returning. I wanted to be close to him. I wanted him.

Paul felt the same. We had bonded in so many ways during this journey. Before we even got out of the car, we were in each other's arms. I couldn't stop the feeling. We didn't have any condoms, and I surely didn't want to get pregnant. We kind of pushed the speed limit to the nearest grocery store. I patiently waited in the car, and eagerly looked for him each time the exit door opened. It seemed as if he was gone forever.

Then we *raced* home and ended up in his bed. The passion was delightful, better than the high from ice water, better than the swimming pool days!

I was still a virgin at thirty and didn't have any experience in the bedroom. I had always felt left out and terribly naive, but after this experience, I was a new woman.

Paul was gentle, tender, loving, and wanted to please me. It was all about me first — my needs and fulfillment. It wasn't like our early, unpleasant, encounters, which didn't involve intercourse. This was something very new and beautiful. I didn't think I would know what to do, but with Paul, lovemaking came naturally. And like any other favorable change in my life, I wanted to do it over and over again. I couldn't get enough sex, affection, and his tender arms around me. The urges in the swimming pool could not be compared to being with a man, especially one that I loved.

I looked forward to climbing into bed each night or experiencing an afternoon delight. I was making up for lost time. He said I was keeping him young. Paul made me feel like a natural woman, and the physical intimacy continued. It became a source of enormous pleasure for me.

I overheated during sex; that hadn't changed. Paul bought the biggest fan he could find. It helped considerably. I waited until I felt cool before getting out of bed. I can't imagine any man allowing a huge box fan to be blowing directly on him, in the middle of winter, while having sex. And in the summer, I added an oscillating floor fan and an air conditioner. It didn't bother Paul. Whatever I needed was okay with him.

It wasn't my style to use moderation. Soon, I expected sex every night before going to sleep. Then sex became an obsession. Probably, most men wouldn't mind that. In general, Paul was very accommodating. He enjoyed our active sex life; however, some evenings, after working ten or twelve hours in the ninety-degree heat using a jackhammer or pick and shovel, not even Viagra would have helped. Paul wanted to go to sleep. No, he needed to go to sleep.

I tossed and turned for what seemed to be hours. All I could think about was how wonderful I slept after sex. So, in the typical manner that I rationalized my existence, I came to the conclusion sex was as good as a sleeping pill. Without it, I couldn't sleep. Even when I wasn't in the mood, I believed I still had to have sex, and it became another daily phobia. In time, I realized if I relaxed and put my mind in a peaceful setting with calming thoughts, I eventually fell asleep.

Paul worried about me constantly, and at the same time, it made him feel needed. I enjoyed being with him and doing what I could to brighten his day. After his evening bath, I gave him a rubdown, which eased his sore and knotted physique after a hard day in construction. I enjoyed touching his warm body and feeling the firm muscles. It was relaxing for me, too. And these times gave us quiet moments together. Often, he commented that he could have never kept going each day without the rubdowns. Then I knew he needed me, too.

I was losing weight gradually, and my body was forming curves in all the right places. A new, fashionable wardrobe was much needed.

Most materials overheated me. I had no interest in shopping; however, Paul convinced me to go window-shopping. I was about ready to give up when we detoured into a small shop where incense and candles were burning. I had never seen so much silver and turquoise jewelry. I told him it wasn't a place to look for clothes, but he insisted. On a rack off to the side, Paul found a few stylish garments. A mauve, wraparound, polyester skirt and matching camisole top caught my eye. It draped well on my figure. It also made me look a little slimmer. There were two of the same shops in the area, and we continued to buy the same outfit until they were out of stock. A few other shops sold a similar skirt. Paul washed them over and over again in hopes the fabric would eventually soften and become thinner and feel okay next to my skin. They didn't. We finally gave up and found a seamstress to copy the skirt.

The first skirt was a trial. Once I was sure of the material not overheating me, I had the seamstress make several in various colors. I wore the same style daily, and it brought about a uniform look. The sameness didn't bother me; comfort was the priority. I also wore a little makeup and put on a sparkle or two. I wanted Paul to take a second look. He commented regularly. What woman doesn't enjoy that? Life was heading in a good direction.

Paul bought me clothes or fabric, jewelry, pocketbooks, several scarves, hats, and gloves. When I showed a hint of interest, he bought it, if our income allowed it. I thought he should treat himself more, but all I heard again and again was "I want you to look nice."

I had a terrible time with hemorrhoids. They bled excessively; so much so I had to wear a sanitary napkin. I also sat in cold water to shrink them and then applied Vaseline. At times, the ointment stained my skirts. Paul never let me leave the house with a stain in my skirt, even if it was barely noticeable. He thought my image, or first impression, was a reflection of who I was. He told me I was beautiful, and soiled clothing was a big takeaway.

On weekends, or when Paul was laid off, he joined me at McDonald's or wherever I ended up eating my dinner. With both of us eating out, it once again became too expensive. I cooked our dinner, and Paul ate at home. Then we left for a restaurant, and I had my dinner.

As normal as I was beginning to feel, we were the odd couple that arrived at McDonald's, Long John Silver's, or Pizza Hut every day at the *same* time and sat in the *same* booth. We had checked out the dining room upon our first visit to each place. Normally, the table with the most moving air was by a window and the farthest from the hot kitchen.

We were totally opposite in stature. Paul was short and usually a little stout; if he was working for one particular company we called the workout camp, then he was trim. He thoroughly enjoyed eating. He could easily sit down to a meal anytime of the day or start over after finishing one. I was tall and thin and avoided consuming too many calories. I lugged around a huge, canvas, beach bag filled with food.

We only ordered drinks, and we sat in the restaurant for, at least, an hour. The process took a long time because I didn't just sit and eat. I drank an iced, diet soda first. Then I sat for about fifteen minutes waiting for my body to be cool enough to eat. Sitting in a cool spot and drinking a cold liquid took the place of using cold water. During the winter months, the combination of a cold drink and sitting in the cold turned my fingers white. My fingers hurt until the circulation came back, but other than that, I didn't realize the seriousness of what was happening to my hands.

I ate my dinner in a specific order, and the process never changed. I started my meal with a bag of cold vegetables. Next, I ate the main entrée and a hot vegetable along with a cold, diet soda. Last came fruit, yogurt, and hot coffee. Paul drank coffee and read the paper. I was obsessed with the exactness of the entire process — from the time I left the house until I finished my meal.

Paul could read lips, and it wasn't long before he knew what people were talking about. He was very observant and was able to pick up on the snickering and whispering. I didn't even think about my behavior.

Later, Paul told me what he witnessed. Other people, according to Paul, thought I was weird. It didn't upset me. The only thing that mattered was eating where the temperature was satisfactory and eating enough to stay healthy. The rest was nothing.

I was very sensitive to the airflow in every restaurant. If, for some reason, it diminished, I knew it immediately. I complained throughout the entire meal either to Paul or to the management. I gave up cold water in order to eat, but I replaced it with cool, moving air. I would move heaven and earth to get what I needed. Finding a chilly restaurant was sometimes exhausting. Generally, if I arrived at my usual eatery early, the table where I always sat was available. Occasionally, I was late, and it was occupied. I became upset, then impatient, and couldn't eat until the party vacated. Once it was available, I quickly moved my belongings to the desired table.

The cool air blew down over my body, and the heat evaporated. The taste buds were enlightened, and dinner began. Most people probably don't even consider anything like this, especially in winter. It was on my mind all the time.

Long John Silver's was only satisfactory in the summer. If it wasn't, I complained and asked them to turn up the air-conditioning. One manager usually complied and was very nice about it. Then a new fellow was hired. He was conscious about saving energy, and he completely ignored me. I left and never returned. I alternated between two McDonald's restaurants, choosing whichever was the coolest.

Eventually, I chilled my core temperature down so far that I craved *very hot liquids*. My body must have been telling me something: living in too much cold air. I insisted on extremely hot tea or coffee. I usually didn't wait for the liquid to cool. I couldn't wait to get the drink in my stomach. In doing so, I burned the roof of my mouth over and over again. The skin peeled off in one large sheet. This went on for years until, one day, I burned the upper back part of my mouth so badly I decided to have my dentist take a look. He said my mouth was all right, even though it was severely burned, but to be more careful in the future. It didn't heal for months, and I still have a scar from that incident. At times, learning the hard way was my downfall.

On occasion, Paul and I had words over eating out at the *same* place day after day. The struggle of finding cool air was tiring. Paul repeatedly suggested I eat at home, but I refused. Tempers flared, words were said, tears were shed, and then there were long periods of silence. The quiet was worse than the words. In the mind, the chain of events snowballed and became more stressful than the original issue.

Paul wanted me to change. I wouldn't budge from this daily jaunt.

Sometimes Paul commented, "You don't love me enough. If you did, you would change."

When I was going through this unpleasant time in my life, that kind of statement from him only saddened me. Loving Paul was one thing; giving up an obsessive-compulsive behavior was a different matter. In my way of thinking, the two could not be linked together. It was easy to love Paul. It was not easy to give up what I believed to be a physical need for survival. Without life, there would be no *me* to love Paul.

Even if I could have stopped my obsessions on the spot, this amazing journey would not have been as meaningful. Our love grew stronger because of what we went through. My experiences, good and bad, created a stronger woman. I believe everything happens for a reason — even the suffering.

Over the years, we had similar moments and demonstrations with various other subjects. When I first met Paul, if something really upset him, which was usually related to his work in construction, I also felt the brunt of it. At that point in time, I was never sure if I would be staying or leaving. I had never shared my life with a man until I met Paul. I didn't have any experience with relationships. During the unpleasant disagreements, I was sure life would never be the same, and our love for each other would perish.

The longer I was with him, the more I understood it wasn't me. Every day can't be perfect. I was judging the moment without knowing the underlying issues. We never truly know what is going on in another person's mind. My fear of his occasional unpleasant disposition went away, and I knew I would always have a home with him someplace. I wasn't really the problem, even though I thought I was at the time. Our love for each other always brought us back on track.

I didn't like feeling sad and upset, especially when I really liked the person I was fighting with. During those unpleasant sessions, I found it even more difficult to eat. My body became so warm I couldn't keep my skin cool no matter what I did. I was close to feeling cool, unpleasant words were said, and then I'd be hot all over again.

When I first started eating out in restaurants, I was high on the idea of what I had accomplished — given my history of how I used to go about eating my meals. As the years moved along, obtaining the right conditions became more difficult. That same complaint was eminent when I was swimming. The more Paul and I expected cold temperatures, the more disappointed we were. Possibly, a spiritual energy was trying to tell me something.

At times, Paul said, "Let's try a different restaurant. Maybe we'll have better luck elsewhere."

My immediate reply was a flat-out *no*. Then as I thought about it, I felt bad he had to endure this daily drudgery. I wanted to make him happy, and I agreed. By the time we found a suitable restaurant, I wished we hadn't. The nerve-racking, upsetting, and irritating drive around the Capital District was past disturbing. Thinking negatively before we even started didn't help the tension, and more times than not, I developed a migraine.

In every restaurant, I asked the hostess where the coldest section was located. Not trusting her judgment, I went from one table to the next and stood, waiting to feel the cold air. In many restaurants, there was only one table that had adequate moving cool air. If I thought the air temperature was sufficient, I actually sat at the table to test it out. Paul always thought it was fine and was ready to order. The waitress patiently waited while I took forever to make up my mind.

Paul explained to the waitress, "She needs it very cool so she can eat."

Then I became annoyed; I felt I was being rushed. Paul was patient up to a point. I would tell him the restaurant was fine, and then I'd change my mind. After much deliberation, the evening was spoiled anyway.

The staff looked at us like we were *wacky*.

We picked up all our gear, walked out, and tried another restaurant — and another and another. By the time we found one, neither of us was able to enjoy our dinner. Our mood drastically changed, and silence and tension prevailed.

Ever since I was a young adult, negative conversation affected my appetite. Unfortunately, I carried this baggage with me for years. It was, and is, a fear. Forty years later, I'm better, but I don't welcome it.

Over and over, I told Paul I needed a guarantee. Searching elsewhere for the right temperature was aggravating and caused too much stress. The usual place I went each day was all I needed. Paul said there were no guarantees in life except taxes and death and his love for me.

I didn't socialize much. Searching for the perfect temperature was close to impossible, plus it overtaxed my body and took away the pleasure of the day.

I missed being around people. Slowly, I began to let go of the rein I held so tight. I signed up for a makeup course at the local high school. It was only a few short sessions in the evening, which worked out perfectly with the rest of my routine. After making the commitment, I wasn't sure I'd be able to attend. As it turned out though, it was early spring, and the outdoor temperature was moderate, as was the classroom. It was nice to be with other women and out of the house on my own. And best of all, I was able to tolerate my surroundings. Every morning thereafter, for almost twenty-four years, I was eager to practice what I learned, and when I viewed myself in the mirror, I was glad I grabbed the opportunity.

The camera Paul bought me was more complicated than any camera I ever owned; therefore, I attempted a photography course at a local university. The parking lot seemed to be miles away from the building. By the time I arrived in the classroom, I was sizzling. I couldn't concentrate or cool down. I never finished the course.

I felt the need to walk after every meal, especially after dinner. It became an obsessive cooling process, an alternative to swimming. At the mall, I didn't always walk where everyone else did. Most of the time, it wasn't a comfortable temperature; whereas, one of the department stores inside the mall was perfect. We walked within one small section of the store for close to an hour — around and around and around. The salespeople asked if we needed help.

Paul said, "No, we're just walking; she needs to walk to stay cool."

From the looks we received, it was obvious what their assessment was. Their world and ours was far from the same.

Paul's children gathered together at their mother's house for Christmas dinner. Paul and I were always invited, which made me feel as if I were part of the family. I sat off to the side while they all ate dinner. Some holidays were quite warm, and they even opened a window for me so I wouldn't overheat. After Paul finished eating, he went with me to a restaurant. I ordered a meal, but I always brought along hot and cold vegetables, fruit, and my own bread. It didn't matter if the restaurant was the classiest place in town; I still lugged my huge, canvas bag around with me.

Paul always said, "Don't be embarrassed because you brought along some items to enhance your meal. Put the bag of vegetables right up on the table and enjoy your dinner."

After a few years, Paul and I eliminated the family gatherings and only dined at a restaurant.

Even in ice storms or blizzards, *we went through just like the mailman.* On holidays, we couldn't walk in the malls because they were closed; therefore, we searched for whatever was open. One year, we went to the local airport. At least, we had a lot of space and no people. At the time, the airport hadn't gone international. It was rather intimidating not seeing anyone but the staff, but nice to have the freedom.

Very few restaurants are open on Christmas Day. I wouldn't eat at home, and it was almost impossible to find an eatery serving dinner. There was one Christmas I will never forget. It was bitter cold, and the temperature was dangerously low. Even the restaurants usually open on this holiday were closed due to the weather. We found one open, about fifteen minutes from the house. The day produced a blizzard like no other, and the visibility was very poor. Paul was very hesitant. I was positive we'd be fine. He was always worried about my body temperature and what we would do if the car broke down. The weather station said the wind chill was fifty below zero and people should stay at home. Safety wasn't on my mind, only being able to eat and then walk after dinner.

As luck would have it, no other cars were on the road. They were smarter than we were. I could feel the tension between us, yet Paul didn't complain. If I had to travel in such horrendous conditions, he wasn't about to let me go alone. The roads were slippery. I held the wheel tight and prayed the car would stay where it belonged. The wipers had a difficult time, even on high, as the snow clung in chunks to the blade. The windows steamed up, and visibility was close to nil. Occasionally, the car slid, and I held my breath and prayed. The distance seemed to be much longer than I remembered. We finally made it in one piece.

The meal was all right, but due to the circumstances, we weren't relaxed. Paul was anxious to get home before the night closed in on us. I wanted to do *my thing* and walk in a mall just like I always did. There was nowhere to walk close by, and the roads were much too dangerous to go anywhere but home. Paul suggested I walk in the coatroom. I complained it was way too small, but he said there were no other options. I paced back and forth many times. It wasn't long before an employee entered.

He approached us with an unpleasant look and said, "Please, stop walking; you are scaring the customers."

Paul told me to walk until I was ready to quit.

Chapter 17
Out of the Deep Freeze

I depended on Paul to fix whatever needed fixing. He made each day okay. Whatever obstacle I encountered, he tried to help me conquer it. If an item could be purchased, Paul bought what I needed, within limits, of course.

Unfortunately, the biggest job was to overcome the heat I felt, and only I could accomplish that. And if I were blessed, someday it would disappear.

I had stopped using ice cubes and ice water in the bathtub long ago. The need for *extreme* cold was decreasing. I welcomed some warmth only if I knew there was a guaranteed way of lessening it if need be. So far, walking was significant, followed by a multitude of huge box fans, air-conditioning, cool sponge baths, and the type of food I consumed. With so many fans in the house, we had trouble finding enough storage space in the winter.

When the brisk, cool days of October arrived, I knew it wouldn't be long before the furnace was humming. That only meant one thing: a warm house. I dreaded the fall season for many reasons. It was during the fall when I usually became very ill and was frequently hospitalized. Finding cool, moving, indoor air was close to impossible. When I added layers of clothes, I felt trapped and unable to sit for long periods of time. The heating system in Paul's house was forced air. No matter where I sat, I felt warm air blowing on me. I felt as if I were fighting an unsolvable predicament.

There was a time when I walked the streets at all hours in order to get away from the uncomfortable warmth. I had always found one way or another to survive. I believe Girl Scout camp had something to do with my survival techniques. I was taught to think for myself and believe I could overcome any unpleasant situation. That doesn't mean I functioned fully with the uncomfortable heat. And I didn't panic either. I learned how to cope with it one way or another.

Instead of suffering all the time, I came up with alternatives to lessen the discomfort. We bought several small, electric, floor heaters so the furnace didn't run all the time. I could tolerate summer fans pushing around the warm air but not the warm air coming from the furnace in the wintertime. Go figure.

In the summer, we had big fans in every room of the house. And there was an air conditioner pumping out cold air in the bedroom. I put a fan in the kitchen window adjacent to where I sat for a meal. The location was all right in eighty-or ninety-degree weather. However, the fan stayed in the window all year long.

During the winter months, without fail, the furnace kicked on as soon as I was ready to eat. A nice, cool sponge bath had just been completed. My taste buds were turned on, and I anticipated a nice, big breakfast. And then the heat poured out of the floor register. It quickly made its way to my body, overtaking the coolness and leaving me helpless of a reversal. Aggravation and lack of control followed. The window fan helped counteract the furnace heat. Sometimes, I had to remove the snow from the windowsill in order to put the fan in the window.

I was never satisfied with a little cold. I increased it to disastrous proportions. Whenever I drastically chilled my body, the blood left my fingers. The loss of color happened over and over again. This routine was lowering my body temperature. It also increased the risk of Raynaud's syndrome. I didn't like temperature change, yet I was creating a drastic one. Low body temperature resulted in horrific, painful migraines, which led to vomiting and, at least, seventeen hours of bed rest, and it wasn't restful at all.

Finally, I realized I had to put a stop to this behavior. I propped the fan up to the window, just not *in* the window. During the course of several weeks, I closed the window a fraction each day. At last, I managed with the window closed. I still used a fan, but it was warm air instead of the frigid, outdoor air.

I had a thirst for companionship and being around people. The home aides filled this void. I would have been fine without them except for conversation in the morning prior to bathing. Fear held me back on dismissing them. Once they were gone, I wouldn't be able to get them reinstated; I wasn't sure I was ready for that.

Progress gave me the confidence I could do more and more with my life. I had this wild idea to go back to college. Classes and studies would be a very big challenge and, definitely, a change in my daily routine. I was still battling with temperature changes on all levels *and* a low body temperature. I wanted to attend college and be mentally challenged. I thought I could overcome some of my issues and accomplish this aspiration.

It was a risky decision, and after considering all the advantages, we decided to apply. I say we, not that Paul applied, because he was with me throughout all my adventures. Paul's outlook leaned more toward interaction with people and the companionship. I, on the other hand, also wanted the same; but more importantly, I was looking to extend my education for a better tomorrow. I enrolled, and I was accepted. My father paid for my books, and I obtained a student loan from the government for the college tuition. Everything was in order. I felt young again and vibrantly excited.

The first day of school was a warm, balmy day. The college was in the city, which was much warmer than the village of Latham. The classroom was filled with students. I sat in the back row. Once everyone was seated and the door closed, the heat began to escalate. I felt nauseous and dizzy. The more I attempted to comprehend what the professor was saying, the more my head pounded from the heat. The pressure on my temples was too much. Soon, the heat took over my entire body, and I couldn't focus. I stood up and quickly exited. In my gut, there was a feeling that told me I wasn't ready. At that point, I knew the first day was also my last day at college.

The idea of school was more practical than the reality of it. I felt I had let Paul down and, once again, my father. I was so sure I would be able to endure some heat. It worked at home but not in the classroom. I wasn't living in the deep freeze anymore, yet I learned rather quickly I wasn't healed as much as I thought I was.

Confinement was always very difficult. Being trapped in heat put me in a *panic* state of mind. To sit in one spot or stand in line wasn't my forte. When we went to a doctor's office, I paced up and down the room until my name was called. At the grocery store, I walked around the store while Paul stood in line. When I went shopping alone, I'd pick the shortest checkout line and hope for the best. When the line didn't move quickly, I took long, deep breaths and prayed. As the warmth engulfed my body, my breathing became heavier. When I couldn't take it anymore, I walked out the door, leaving the groceries on the belt.

I made considerable progress over the years, but most of the time, Paul was doing the errands outside the home. I could make myself do it, although I suffered afterward with dreadful migraines. Now, if the entire outdoors had a bubble over it and the inside of it consisted of an even temperature, I'd be fine. That perfect condition is almost impossible, but who knows, with global warming, cities may be covered with domes someday.

I was gradually moving away from the frigid cold. But I had a need for some coolness, which meant Paul and I had to take my body temperature often. I had thermometers in the bedrooms, my pocketbook, the bathrooms, and in the car.

As soon as I didn't look right, Paul said, "Take your temperature."

The signs of low body temperature were an inability to navigate my body, feeling way too warm when the room was cold, excruciating migraines, pale complexion, altered speech, or a spaced-out look. Then we knew it was time to put the thermometer in my mouth. Many times, my body temperature dropped to ninety-two degrees. Then I drank a very warm liquid, took a hot bath, or went under the covers to trap as much heat as possible.

I didn't always acknowledge what was happening. Paul had been with me long enough to see the signs. He quickly brought it to my attention to take action. I will probably have to do this for the rest of my life. Paul's body was always warm; he naturally radiates heat. He was a nice, big, heating blanket. Most of the time, when he held me, my body temperature made its way back up. My loss of body heat happened so often that he always worried about me when we were apart.

Paul often said I should live in a bubble with controlled temperatures. We came close in our home. Unfortunately, as soon as I stepped out of our *home bubble*," and someone wasn't paying attention or watching me, before long, I was in trouble. Attributing factors were inappropriate clothing, not enough carbohyrates, and cold air. All these things were dangerous elements, and I was the last to see what was happening.

Since I started losing weight, I was using artificial sweeteners — and a lot of them. I put the sweetener in yogurt, drinks, on fruit, and in coffee. After dinner, I had coffee and apples. I loved apples. It wasn't enough that I added the sweeteners in my coffee; I also dipped slices of apples in the imitation sweetener. After a meal, there were probably a dozen or more empty wrappers scattered around my coffee cup.

At this particular time in our lives, Paul saw my temperature lingering on the low side, my hands were always turning white, I wasn't thinking clearly, and my speech wasn't clear. He insisted I stop using artificial sweeteners and replace it with table sugar.

This change played a huge role in elevating my body temperature. Of course, I wasn't going to eat sugar all day long; but when it was needed, the real sugar definitely helped.

Time, faith, and Paul were instrumental in the healing process. I was being given the *time* to heal at my own pace. I didn't pray for a kind man to come into my life, yet I know God brought me to *Paul*. And soon, my *faith* would be a part of everyday life.

Paul loved me just the way I was. He certainly gave me time to move forward in my life. I wonder how many men would have put up with me as much as he has over the years. I certainly tested his patience over and over. He believed in what I said; however, he didn't always understand. Even so, he tried to acknowledge and feel the pain I was in. I would say that 98 percent of the time he went along with my obsessions and needs.

Paul recognized the danger signs. He was never sure if what I was doing would help me or hurt me. Nevertheless, he knew from past experiences I balked at any of his suggestions so, most generally, he let me work through it all on my own. Regrettably, it took me a long time to distinguish between destructive and beneficial behavior. I was the last to know.

The beneficial changes that occurred in my life usually came about through drastic measures. I resisted change as along as possible. For survival reasons, my body couldn't take the punishment I was putting it through. Only at that moment, did I realize the change was for the better. When I had no choice but to stop what I was doing, and I was forced to make a change, then I allowed change in my routines.

Maybe it was meant to be a slow process. Then I could see how my life was being given back to me. Each change opened a new door. On the other side of the door, I received more out of life — all of which I had lost in the addiction to ice-cold water.

Aiming for total wellness was painful for both of us, but our love grew stronger each year. We were fighting this fight together. I knew he was always with me, forever and always, no matter what. We had our disagreements and small fights from time to time.

It was as if we lived for each other. Overcoming the obstacles together strengthened our relationship. As my addiction weakened and the fears lessened, we talked about the progress and said, "Remember the ol' days. We don't want to go back there, do we?"

Taking small steps each day, we moved forward — out of the darkness and toward the light.

Paul and I were living in our own world and had very little contact with my family. The bond, I once enjoyed with my family, disappeared during my unpleasant years. I had made some bad choices. And I acted inappropriately. At the time, I blamed my condition, which was only partially to blame, because we all have a choice. At times, I made the wrong ones. These were mistake-filled years. I couldn't go back and live them over again, but I did ask God for forgiveness.

I believe my prayers were answered.

Chapter 18
Reuniting with Dad

All the visits we made to Copake had been brief. There wasn't much conversation. A quick hello, and then Paul and I were out the door, heading back to Latham.

Dad started traveling to and from Saratoga with his racehorse. Paul and I were along the way. I made sure no one came to our house in the morning except the home aide. I didn't want anyone to see, or know of, my bathing routine, certainly not Dad. When he called and asked if it was all right to come by and say hello, I had hoped to be further along in my healing. The day of his first visit, I was extremely nervous. I wasn't sure what time he would arrive. I definitely wanted him to see *normal*. My past had been anything but normal. When he arrived, I didn't want him to see any part of my obsessive behavior. I suggested the time of day, so his visit fit into my routine. I was relieved when he agreed; by then, my breakfast and lunch would be finished. As false as the scene was, I was able to relax.

Paul's home wasn't at all like Dad's house. It was very modest and in need of much repair, but I did what I could to enhance our surroundings, and we were happy.

Each time Dad stopped to see us, we never talked of my addiction or the past. We just spent a little time together, which was nice. I always looked forward to seeing him. He seemed to have changed and was trying to reconnect. I think the horses allowed him to focus on the now. Their special characteristics minimized his stress. He had been around horses on and off his whole life; as a child, he rode Western, and when I was young, we had horses. He seemed to be very proud of what he had accomplished with this new interest. They didn't win all that much; I just think he enjoyed all that went with owning a horse.

Dad knew how much I loved apples. When they were in season, he brought us a bushel of Macouns, my favorite variety. When I saw him coming down the driveway with the apple basket, I knew immediately what they were. It was difficult to stop the memories and the emotions. Our reunion seemed to wash away the unpleasant past. It was just good to be near him and have him back in my life. Even though our visits were brief, we were once again connecting with each other. He took time out of his day to stop and say hello. These moments were a special gift.

My father invited Paul and I to the track when one of his horses was running. Dad's horse won the race, and I had my picture taken with both of them in the winner's circle at Saratoga Raceway.

Our relationship was moving in a positive direction. My father was able to see a glimpse of my improvement. Upon each visit, I became more relaxed and wished he would stop in more often. I looked forward to his *detour* when he was on route to the track; we exchanged what was happening in our lives.

Then Dad stopped coming. He had taken ill, and soon after that, he died.

Both my parents had passed at a young age. I was recovering and making a comeback in life. They were gone from this earth; however, on many a day, I felt as if their spirits were watching and observing my progress. Friends and relatives also made this same statement.

I was blessed to have had these special moments with him.

Chapter 19
Scientific Ward

Albany Medical Center set up a special ward with only eighteen beds for patients with severe medical conditions. In 1981, Dr. Howard asked if I would consider coming into the ward. She and her staff wanted to observe and monitor my daily routine. She also wanted me off sugar and on a restricted diet. Next, they would increase the sugar and caloric intake in my diet. The results would be documented.

I wasn't thrilled about the confinement or going into the hospital while I was feeling good. I had never been admitted under those conditions.

Paul encouraged me to comply. He said if the doctors could help me get better, it would be worth a little bit of inconvenience.

I wanted someone to tell me I could conduct myself in the hospital the same as I did at home. To, at least, be able to take sponge baths, if I needed to, prior to eating and have the freedom to walk. I had so much fear swelling inside of me; it was difficult to make a sensible evaluation.

Finally, I agreed. Dr. Howard told me to bring something to occupy my time. She suggested a drawing tablet and pencil.

The night before I left, I was on edge and sleepless. I was afraid I had made the wrong decision. I had a good routine going on at home and in the fast food restaurants. A change like this, even for a short time, was scary. I was in the habit of a light beer during dinner, which enhanced my appetite and helped me to relax. I even tried to picture myself in the room eating without cool, moving air or the beer. Then fear made me question my ability. As a safety net, I actually packed one beer. No one ever knew about it, not even Paul. And I brought along a miniature, battery-operated fan.

As Paul and I walked into the room where I would be sleeping, I took one look and burst into tears. The room was ugly and depressing. There was this big, plastic tent around the other bed with a huge, green rubber hand sticking out of the plastic. My description probably doesn't sound all that terrible; however, the entire scene had a depressing look about it.

I said to Paul, "Don't make me stay; it's awful, and it's so hot in here. I won't be able to sleep or eat. I'll never make it."

Paul hugged me and said, "It's not so bad. Don't even look at it. Just be happy it has nothing to do with you, and focus on being a scientific case. That's special."

He kept saying, "You'll make it. I know you will. You can do it. It's only for a short time. Once you are here, you'll adjust; you always do. I can't make you stay; it's up to you. It's your choice. All I can do is make it as pleasant as possible. First, maybe we can get rid of that big, green hand."

Ironically, my fear became a joke between us. From time to time, we said, "Remember the big, green, ugly hand in the scientific ward?" And then we laughed.

After Paul left, I went to the coffee shop and purchased bouillon, juice, and a cheese sandwich. I wasn't hungry at all. Crying always made me especially warm, which, in turn, took away my appetite.

Paul arrived at the *crack of dawn* the next morning. His plan was to fix something special or anything I might want to eat. We had a small refrigerator in the room plus full use of the kitchen in the ward. He brought in special meats, fish, garlic, potatoes, vegetables, and cooking wine. He sautéed in garlic, and the aroma was unbelievable. The entire ward was overcome with the magnificent smells of his cooking.

The nurses joked with us, and one asked, "Okay, what's on the menu for today?"

The staff went out of their way to be extremely pleasant. They made the stay a lot easier. I had a great deal of freedom; I liked that part. I could eat in my room or go down to the cafeteria or coffee shop as long as I told them what I ate. I was allowed to walk anywhere within the hospital or walk the grounds, as long as I let them know my whereabouts. It was April; the air was balmy and just beautiful to be outdoors.

Paul bought me a portable radio to bring to the hospital. As I changed the stations, I heard a great song, "Morning Train," by Sheena Easton. It reminded me of Paul going to work, working hard all day, and coming home to me at night. The beat, the words, and the tune were perfect. "Morning Train" became our song. Thereafter, every time it came on the radio, we turned up the volume, closed our eyes, and smiled in between singing along.

I was even allowed to leave the hospital as long as nothing was scheduled. One afternoon, as we were signing out, the head nurse winked at Paul and knew why we were leaving. We drove home to make love. I could have stayed lost in his arms for the rest of the day. I returned to the hospital renewed and glowing.

When we checked back in, the head nurse said, "Did you have a good time?"

Blushing, I said, "Oh, yes, we had a very enjoyable ride. The sun is excessively warm today."

I believe the staff knew better.

My room had a corkboard, perfect for greeting cards. One, in particular, was my favorite: a bear with his head in a honey pot. Lying in bed with nothing to do, I stared at this card frequently. Dr. Howard had said to bring along a sketchpad for a reason. And here was the reason right in front of me. I began to sketch one card after another.

This was the beginning of my *art period*. I was doing something very creative. And it looked pretty darn good. I went to sleep feeling like I had a purpose in life, instead of thinking about medical. I knew I still had health problems, but this was progress and a great diversion. Drawing was something I wanted to pursue further once I left the hospital. I was too excited about the results to stop now.

Paul was very impressed when he came into my room the next morning. He liked what he saw and encouraged me to continue. The repetition of his praise certainly boosted my confidence. He returned the following day with lots of brightly colored markers. Paul believed in having the right tools for any job; they were a vital part of a person's progress. His idea worked.

Little did I know I was about to reawaken a passion I had as a teen: my love of drawing. When I graduated from high school, I had only just begun to touch the surface, and then the drawing stopped. Now, I just might be able to develop it further. This new activity began because of a special doctor, Dr. Howard. Something or someone triggered this new endeavor. Maybe a guardian angel was sitting on her shoulder, whispering in her ear on my behalf.

Dr. Howard came in daily to tell me how the study was going. She informed me of a thesis she was writing on my case. Maybe this study would clarify some questions and provide some answers for all of us.

Years of not eating sufficiently could have caused a slight stroke and left a lesion in the base of my brain. Anorexia patients can be left with a lifetime of such scars. And there was still the question of which came first. Did I have a pre-existing medical condition that caused me to feel hot or an imbalance that prevented my utilizing calories properly? Or did I develop medical problems as a result of my abuses on my body caused by my obsessive-compulsive behavior? This study could prove a medical case over a psychiatric one.

The study could not be totally documented as planned, because I didn't comply with their regimen. They wanted me to eat too much sugar or none at all. Such an event would only happen when I chose to indulge or when my body gave me the signs. When anyone asked me to change my eating habits, it never happened. I was a stubborn lady when it came to food.

The study ended after two weeks, and I was discharged from the hospital. I thought it turned out to be a good hospital stay. Paul thought it was a waste of time and nothing was accomplished. My blood, vital signs, and body temperature were fine; those readings are common for everyone.

I was finding a way to exist, which was satisfactory to me. I didn't want to alter the process at all. I was afraid to do what was asked. I felt my life was balanced. I was right where I wanted to be, at least, for now. When it was time to move forward, I would know it. I wasn't even looking for a miracle cure. I was just glad to be going home — back to my comfortable familiar habits.

My doctor did remember what Paul told her, and it was documented.

After several episodes of severe disorientation accompanying hypothermia, her boyfriend removed all foods containing artificial sweeteners and replaced them with foods high in sucrose content.

The complete case report can be found on the Internet at http://www.sciencedirect.com

Chapter 20
The Artist in Me: The Art Period

I left the Scientific Ward very enthused about drawing. Possibly, nothing more was supposed to happen at this particular time — a different kind of prescription.

I had a multitude of compliments while in the hospital; however, Paul was my biggest fan. He was just as excited as I was about my new art venture.

Paul was planning the next day as soon as we left the hospital; buying art supplies was on the agenda. The local art store had a wonderful inventory; too much to pick from. I almost gave myself a headache trying to decide what to buy; however, the massive display was extremely motivating. We always returned to the same art store, and eventually, the employees recognized me as an artist. I was now on a mission with a dream to pursue.

It was grand to be home from the medical center. To some degree, home was a place that sheltered us from many problems, mostly environmental changes and people snickering. A lot of love was housed within the walls. I especially missed Keefer, a real love bug that found his way into our hearts and settled there nicely. In no time at all, we were back into our comfy routine. I felt safe and secure, knowing exactly how the day would play out.

The home aide service had given me good stability in the house, but I felt it was time to discontinue them. The aide only came in the morning, mostly for company. I was still afraid to begin my day without someone in the house, better yet, at the kitchen table. I rehearsed the scene over and over in my mind and how it would play out if I were alone. Paul worked Monday through Friday; that was five days of anxiety. He asked if I was sure I wanted to cancel the aides. I assured him it was okay, even though I hadn't entirely convinced myself.

After my hot bath each morning, the cold sponge bath continued. That daily routine was still very much a necessity. I assumed I'd be spending all my mornings this way for the rest of my life.

For a considerable amount of time, a home aide was with me prior to the sponge bath. Speaking to her just before bathing became part of the obsession. I desperately depended on that security. Subsequently, I moved on to the next phase of my morning, which was eating. Like any habit or addiction, letting her go was a very difficult decision.

After we discontinued the services, I used the telephone to connect to a substitute for the home aide. I called the operator and asked the time of day.

That was a favorite. The next day, the local airport and when a flight was leaving for a city I picked out of the blue. I called a retail store or the library and said I had the wrong number.

I looked through the phone book. Most anyone was sufficient. I only needed to hear a voice for a few seconds. This was the *thing* that worked for me, and it continued longer than it should have. I didn't even tell Paul. I was afraid if I told him, my plan would be jinxed. Most likely, he would get someone to be with me. I knew, in my heart, I would, eventually, be fine with no assistance. I had faith in myself it was possible; it was just going to take time.

I finally confided in Paul.

He said, "I can record my voice, and you can hear me when you need someone."

I needed a live person on the other end. Weird as it was, I believed it.

When the aide left, my hairdresser did too. I was very blessed to find an extraordinary stylist at a nearby salon. She was a beautiful, young gal with a great personality and lots of patience. I looked forward to seeing once a week, and not just for my hair; we became friends. We talked about all the *stuff* women talk about when men aren't around.

I insisted the hairstyle be exactly the same as it had been for many years: hair parted down the middle of my head with two perfect braids — tight, tight, tight — coiled around on top of my head and anchored with bobby pins. My hair stayed in this style until the next appointment. We repeated the same process each week for about five years. With all the hairdressers involved, the same hairdo existed close to eight years. I wore tight braids for so long the right side of my head was void of hair. Even so, I continued to ask my hairdresser/friend to braid it tighter.

When I was scheduled for MRI tests and CAT scans, I was required to remove all the bobby pins. I was more nervous about my hair than the test. The only time my hair was on my neck and down my back was before my stylist washed it. The warmth that was created by my hair made me edgy and irritable; I insisted it be braided immediately. Before scheduling the test, I made sure my friend was working on the same day. As soon as the test was over, I wanted my hair braided, not two hours later. I went directly from point A to point B.

My hair stylist moved to Florida. Finding someone to take her place was more than upsetting; I made it a traumatic situation. She was a good friend and a significant part of my obsession. I felt incomplete and depressed without her. As much as I wanted my friend to change her mind, her dreams were different then mine.

As I worked myself away from my deadly past, I invented ways to help me move forward. I could have chosen liquor or drugs. I didn't. In that respect, I didn't think the phobias were all that bad, although it was still part of an obsessive-compulsive behavior. I convinced myself I needed all my behavior patterns in order to endure life. Each habit or ritual or routine became so embedded in my existence it was like breathing. I was sure each one of them could never be eliminated.

Each workday, Paul drank his couple cups of coffee and then went to work. This time of the day was fresh and new. My hands and brain were ready to work. The crisp, white paper on the drawing board was most appealing in the tranquility of early morning. I set aside about an hour for quieting my soul and putting ideas on paper. Figuring out what to draw, colors to use, perspective — all improved my ability to focus. I cherished this time of the day: quiet and calm, creative and productive. It was a nice blend. The only interruption or distraction was Keefer; and he was easy to tolerate. Once I left the drawing board, my body was in motion, except for mealtime.

Drawing started to fit in nicely with my daily obsessions. For me, this was a serious time to work, so being alone was good. I was putting as much time into drawing as I was staying cool.

I had a variety of brushes, pencils, paint and books — all very helpful for a beginner. Observation and experimentation, and not being afraid to try, were the biggest assets. I was passionate about the creativity, and detail was my forte.

I was surprised by what I saw on paper. I didn't think I had it in me. I was growing and putting a great deal of effort and time into something worthwhile. After each drawing session, whether it was to my satisfaction or a disaster, I was pleased with the time well spent. I started exhibiting my artwork in a few local banks and picked up some individual sales plus commission work. Several small businesses hired me to create signs where I incorporated calligraphy with animation.

One client was very special. She purchased a whimsical painting of teddy bears. Each time she had a newborn baby, I received a telephone call to paint more teddy bears with a similar theme. While sketching her requests, I recalled moments in my childhood. I came up with a slogan I attempted to weave into my future paintings: Art Related to Moments in People's Lives™.

I joined the area art league, which was a nice swing into another element. I looked forward to the first art league meeting. We arrived early, chatted with other artists, and waited for the meeting to begin. It wasn't long before I was overcome with heat, followed by a migraine; we quietly departed, disappointed. Paul and I quickly learned that each building had a different heating system, and there was no consistency. Unfortunately, this factor eliminated my attendance at most social gatherings; however, it didn't discourage the desire to sketch and stay in touch with other artists.

I attempted my own style in acrylics and picked up tips wherever I could. Extra training would have been beneficial and possibly lessened the stressful moments that came from being an inexperienced artist; however, the deep concentration was helpful. I was totally captivated, as if under a spell, when I was at my drawing table. The process of transferring my vision onto the paper was perplexing, but determination and perseverance produced what I was aiming for most of the time.

In 1981, Paul and I came up with two posters for the workplace. One showed the proper way to bend and lift. The other poster promoted hygiene for washrooms with an emphasis on consideration for plumbing problems.

We went to a local printer with four drawings. The anticipation of the finished product on the printer's choice of paper created both excitement and stress. My heart rate was probably off the charts, the day we walked into the office to view the final work. We encountered some minor problems, which were corrected with another run at no charge to us. As I held the finished piece in my hand, I felt chills up my spine. I saw the huge stacks of brown paper packages, and it took a moment to sink in that it was all my artwork. We were more than ready for orders.

There were several businesses we contacted, with our major *hopeful* being the State of New York. We patiently waited for the purchase order to be delivered. The New York State Office of General Services was our first big sale. Other local orders included Pizza Hut, Taconic Telephone Company, and Regal Press.

Years later, in 1987, New York State commissioned me to do a poster for a large renovation project. The Twin Towers in New York City was one of the buildings under construction at the time. I felt as if I were stepping up a notch when I met with the top man at OGS in Albany, New York. I was a little nervous as I walked into his office but prepared to take on whatever was decided. I left the room somewhat taller, and smiling more than he could see.

Paul and I knew the manager of our local Pizza Hut because we often went there for dinner. During one of our brief conversations, he learned of my artistic ability. I was asked to design an elaborate invitation. It was being sent to the president of the corporation, inviting him to an event at the local franchise. A few weeks later, he presented me with another assignment. He needed a sign and business card for his dog kennel.

The *art period* was a huge stepping-stone on my journey. There were many moments of frustration; I even grew from that. The pay was minimal; that was fine. I was an artist, because I enjoyed the challenge and creativity; and as a huge bonus, if people smiled when viewing my art, then I had accomplished what I had hoped for.

Paul was also inspired by my creativity. I knew he had something on his mind. He was quiet and deep in thought. For several days, while I was eating my dinner, he was jotting words down on a paper napkin. He composed the most beautiful poem, and it was even read by one of our local radio stations.

Turning Point
We were both a drift
Set a cast by life's turmoil,
Not knowing which direction or caring.
Not until the tides came in full,
Did we care enough to seek out life itself.
Now that I have found you I could never let you go.

Paul Vona, 1982

I continued my passion for drawing and, in 1985, was surprisingly rewarded. I received a telephone call from a very prominent woman working for the New York State Office of General Services. She asked if I wanted to participate in a poster contest. The first year, her committee asked a famous illustrator of children's books to draw the poster. The following year, and henceforth, they decided to have an unpublished, local artist. I agreed and went to work with brush in hand. The title of my painting was *Imagination*. I wasn't as blessed as a fellow artist, Fred Gonsowski. His piece won the NYS poster contest one year.

In 1986, the prominent woman from the State asked Fred and me to participate in a fundraiser. She asked me to submit my painting *Imagination*. The event was going to be held at Sotheby's Auction in New York City — an exhibition of paintings by Henry Fonda and a benefit art auction for the Very Special Arts. The proceeds were to benefit the Henry Fonda Young Playwrights Project. She invited both of us to the opening. We were to take the train with her to New York City. This was definitely a new challenge, and a memory of a lifetime. Paul said okay; however, he emphasized all the negatives I might encounter. I went with the positives, and we made plans to go.

The four of us took the train into Grand Central Station, where we hailed a taxi to Sotheby's Auction House. Many actors attended; and others contributed their works: Loretta Swit, George Segal, Peter Max, Peter Falk, Frank Sinatra, Henry Fonda, Ronald Regan, and the Walt Disney Company. I was in awe the whole time I was there. The paintings were marvelous, and the people were intriguing; but the purpose was the most important. The event would go down in history for me, and one none of us would ever forget.

The return trip to Albany wasn't so pleasant. The train didn't have any heat. I was freezing the entire time coming back. I could feel a migraine coming on and couldn't wait to get off the train and hurry home. The following day, all I could remember was the experience of being at Sotheby's, and one of my paintings was on the auction block. There was no need to remember the painful part.

We didn't know if my painting even sold and, if it did, how much it brought. Sadly, we had to leave early in order to catch a train back to Albany. Paul said he didn't want to part with my painting. The next day, he told me he wanted to buy it back if no one bid on it. He called Sotheby's and learned it was still in the auction house. Two days after being in New York City, Paul boarded the train and returned to Sotheby's, ready to put an offer on it.

When he arrived and inquired about my painting, he was told that during the evening of the auction, a woman placed a bid for one hundred dollars. She ended up taking it home. The staff didn't want to give him any more information. Paul wandered around and, in one of the back rooms, found a girl organizing the unsold paintings. He told the employee how much the painting meant to him, and was there anyway to find out who bought *Imagination*? She obtained the information. It was a woman in New Jersey. Paul was able to reach her by telephone. He asked to buy it; but sadly enough, the woman wouldn't accept his offer. She told him she wasn't about to sell it for anything.

Paul did buy two paintings by Fred Gonsowski. They were rather large and cumbersome, but he knew how much I adored Fred's work. He was always trying to make me happy.

After Paul got home, he said, "I could have kicked myself for not buying one of the paintings by Hot Lips!"

He was referring to Hot Lips Houlihan played by Loretta Swit in the M*A*S*H* television series. He always liked her character on the show. I guess the whole experience was rather overwhelming for Paul. I was so proud of him for going to New York City all by himself.

The price of one hundred dollars, for my painting, didn't sound like much at Sotheby's; but to me, the whole adventure was worth a million.

There were fond memories of the bear scenes I painted for the mother-to-be. She was extremely happy when I showed her the finished products. Those thoughts inspired me to sketch more bears. This time, I put a whimsical, country flare within the painting and placed a bear in an old-fashioned bathtub.

Over time, I submitted my artwork to many card companies. The response letter was always the same; we like your work, but we are not interested at this time. Nothing stopped me from trying. I mailed *the bear in the tub* to a company, by the name of Scafa Tornabene, in Nyack, New York. In about two weeks, I received a letter. Paul and I were used to rejections; it started to feel natural. I opened the letter and screamed.

The letter came from the owner of the company. She liked my bear, *but* I needed to fix the areas where she made notations on my drawing. I was on cloud nine but, at the same time, worried. I so wanted to please her. I resubmitted, and she wasn't happy with the rug on the floor. According to her, it was an awful, *yucky* brown, and it didn't match the room décor.

Why did I use that dreary, dull color? What was I thinking? I was heartbroken. I thought I had lost the chance of a lifetime. The owner told me to fix it and make it right. If my revision was suitable, and I wanted the job, she wanted three more bear scenes, all in the bathroom. I sweated over the darn rug. When I finally believed it was what she wanted, I mailed it.

On the day the letter arrived, my heart was in the back of my throat. I wanted to open it; I didn't want to open it. I didn't realize how much stress could develop from looking at an unopened envelope. Slowly, I tore the paper away and slid out the letter. The owner liked the revision. Four paintings of a bear comprised the series: sitting in the bathtub, brushing his teeth, taking a shower, and wearing a distinguishing bathrobe and admiring himself in a full-length mirror. Paul and I couldn't believe it; a company wanted to publish my work.

I finally reached one of my goals. I received only pennies on each one sold. The total sales didn't amount to much; however, being published by a big company was phenomenal. I sent in more sketches, under a new owner, and all were rejected.

This brief moment had been my time to shine, and it had been worth it.

Chapter 21
Life's Ups and Downs

Every normal person, in fact, is only normal on the average. His ego approximates to that of the psychotic in some part or other and to a greater or lesser extent.

Sigmund Freud

I prayed to God for a normal lifestyle. Is it possible to be a normal person? Is anyone normal? That was what I was striving for, or was I?

The eighties were consumed with my *art period*. I felt some transformation into *some* normalcy. However, much of my OCD still existed.

The majority of our life was spent between home, walking in public buildings, and eating in fast food restaurants.

If Paul said it once, he said it a million times, "It is much easier to control the temperatures in your own home."

I still refused to eat at home. I knew I would always find an acceptable eatery. At times, this persistence was stressful. For some, self-induced suffering can still be an acceptable way to live; I was one of them.

We avoided pleasurable outings to most public buildings and even private homes. Where the environmental temperature was good enough initially, it didn't last. I felt hot even though my body really wasn't. After about ten minutes, I developed a headache. The longer I sat, the worse it became, until I ended up with a migraine and a drop in body temperature. Paul watched me suffer on so many excursions and strongly suggested we stop trying to interact with people or attend most functions. He said it wasn't worth it. I wanted to keep trying; he thought it was too much for me to withstand.

As the years moved along, I learned more about my body and its limitations. Whether I was in or out of my home, I practiced alternative ways to counteract the devastating *hot* or the *low body temperature*.

When I was too hot, I ate foods that were labeled nonfat or low fat. When I needed more heat in my body, I chose just the opposite. Ice cream induced a headache most of the time; I avoided it as much as possible.

Normally, when I don't feel well and crave certain foods, my body is giving me a sign: it needs *calories from fat*. And I do well with a *little caffeine*.

Choosing the *appropriate clothing* during the winter helped keep my body temperature stable. All year long, I wore polyesters next to my skin, but in the colder months, I added many other garments of different materials to help trap my body heat.

I wasn't afraid to involve myself in a *project*. This proved to be a positive diversion, which brought me closer to a total healing. And being busy, in a constructive manner, added quality to the day.

The removal of accumulated, negative obsessions couldn't be dispensed with quickly. It took years to get where I was and years to throw them away. I was whittling them down little by little — over time.

The better shape a person is in, the more the temperature goes up when digestion starts. In the seventies, after all the walking and swimming, I was in excellent cardiovascular shape. The fat and sugar from the ham cheese, and ice cream I digested would have made my body work harder to digest it and raise my body temperature. Unfortunately, the severe cold water, eating my meals in cold temperatures, and life in the cold dropped my body temperature.

I loved to *walk*. It was a good replacement for swimming; however, I was afraid to do all my serious walking outdoors. It was reminiscent of my disastrous past. I didn't want to go there for a repeat performance of needing only outdoor air, so I restricted myself to indoors. Now, I was slowly making some alterations in my lifestyle, so I felt it was time to change that, too. Occasionally, on a warm summer day, I walked a short distance outdoors. If that proved to be successful, I increased the time on my next walk.

I went grocery shopping every day after dinner even when I didn't need anything. I cooled as I walked; this was nothing new. The walking began as a pleasant experience but turned into an obsessive-compulsive practice. Even when I wanted to skip a day, I was afraid to. In my mind, the day would not end well if I didn't walk at the grocery store. Over and over, I proclaimed the principal idea behind this was to cool my skin; without it, I would be too warm to go to sleep. Making a trip to the grocery store also made me feel more like a woman with many things on her *to do* list. At the end of the day, I felt I had done something useful.

For many years, I struggled daily. The journey to come back into this world took up a big part of my life. Sometimes my obsessive behavior was a lot of work, but I never once thought of giving up. The perfect star was out there. I just hadn't found it yet.

Prior to living with Paul, I didn't even want to learn about my body. I just lived out the day. As I began to break out of my cocoon, I was slowly being shown more about me than I sometimes wanted to know. As difficult as it was to let go of any obsession, or the cold-water addiction, each positive change gave me a richer and fuller existence.

When God brought me to Paul, he did it up right.

My healing progress was slow. Paul knew it would take time. He was happy with each small or big improvement. Knowing that, I was able to move forward and improve at my own pace without pressure.

Our income was slight, and we had to watch our pennies, but I felt rich in many ways. Paul's divorce was final, and we had fallen in love. The songs on the radio couldn't have been better. My artwork was progressing, Paul was working, and we were doing some decorating. And to top all of that, Keefer completed our little family.

I believe one of the highlights of this period was attending concerts at the local coliseum we called the Tent. It couldn't compare to the size of the newer arenas. There wasn't any air-conditioning, and the stage wasn't spectacular, but the events were outstanding.

One day, I drove up to the Tent. I walked over to the ticket booth and purchased two tickets. I knew if I discussed it with Paul first he would state the negative possibilities, the temperature of the building for one. It was his way of worrying and protecting me from becoming ill. I desperately wanted Paul and me to see a performance. I convinced myself one way or another we were going.

I was eager to tell Paul about the tickets and our evening out on the town. He gladly agreed. I believe he enjoyed seeing me dressed up with my face all aglow. I had one favorite outfit. It was a white, polyester, wraparound skirt; black-and-white stripe, polyester top; and a pair of red, canvas shoes with a cork wedge bottom. It was perfect for a warm, summer night — and a little sexy by the way it clung to my body. I felt very different when I wore this ensemble. It was as if I had walked from one world into another, like Cinderella at the ball.

On the evening of the concert, the air was balmy with a soft warm breeze. The sun was setting, so the heat of the day had become less, which was in my favor. I even enjoyed walking outdoors prior to the show.

Paul was somewhat uncomfortable inside the tent without air-conditioning, and ironically, I was fine. This surprised me. It also showed me I could withstand more heat than I thought. Possibly, this was a sign of better things to come. My diet didn't consist of any fats or sugars, so those items could have explained part of the contentment. Whatever was happening, it seemed hopeful.

We attended several live shows at the Tent. There were many great performers, including Sammy Davis Jr.; Lou Rawls; Tom Jones; Wayne Newton; Janet Jackson, when she was just starting out; and Engelbert Humperdinck. I couldn't believe we were seeing these well-known people and having somewhat of a social life.

One morning, I was at the drawing board, concentrating on the sketch in front of me. The television was mainly for companionship, so the volume was always on low. I was half paying attention until I heard something about positive thinking. I had to listen.

As a child, I only had to cross the street to attend church. I was there in body but never understood what I read in the Bible. The sermons were somewhat dry, and I looked forward to the closing prayer. When I heard this minister, my ears perked up. This guy was good, and I couldn't help myself. His words were extraordinary and meaningful. He was very positive.

What I was hearing made perfect sense. And even with an affliction, if I had a positive outlook, this way of thinking could be beneficial. So why not give it a try?

I said to myself, "This is how I want to live. I want to be a *positive* person."

I felt a new spark of hopefulness and was eager for the next Sunday service. Of course, I was all bubbly and enthusiastic over what I heard on the television. If only I was able to keep this attitude, maybe my life would be even better.

It wasn't so simple convincing Paul. The construction jobs and the people he worked with didn't make this prospect an easy one. I wanted the same feeling for both of us. Maybe in time, it would happen.

Our life together was good. The days were smooth and almost predictable. My daily routine was consistent. Sponge baths with cool water still followed the hot bath, as well as the need for very cool air during meals. I accepted this as my lifestyle for now because the rest of the day was productive. This reasoning gave me peace of mind.

It was the summer of 1985, and the morning heat was escalating. Paul had left for a construction job, and I was home with Keefer. Since Paul had trained Keefer to stay in his own yard, we allowed him to go out every morning. I always checked on him an hour or so later, and normally, he was sitting at the front entrance.

It was one of those perfect days when I felt high on sunshine, and the summer breeze was so sweet and intoxicating that nothing in the world could take my peaceful moment away.

I was putting on my makeup and singing along to a fantastic song on the radio. The day was calm and heavenly until I heard the doorbell ring. I thought it was odd; rarely, did anyone come to visit early in the morning. I had a very bad feeling as I went down the stairs. A young girl was standing at the front door.

She said, "I think your cat just got hit by a car."

I totally freaked out. The blood rushed to my head, fear set in, I pushed open the door, and ran out screaming into the street. There was my Keefer, lying in the middle of the road with blood all around him. My heart sank, and I couldn't stop crying. I didn't know what to do: if I should hold Keefer, or how to comfort him.

I said over and over, "Dear, Lord, please don't let my Keefer die." But I was almost positive he was gone.

The girl got a flat piece of cardboard. I carefully laid him on it and then rushed to my car. With a river of tears streaming down my cheeks, so much so I could hardly see to drive, we rushed Keefer to the nearest veterinarian. All the while, I was hoping and praying he just might still be alive. I gave him to the girl at the front desk and waited in fear for the outcome. When the doctor returned, I knew the answer. I was in shock and could hardly move. It felt like someone just knocked the wind out of me, and I wished this were all a bad dream.

I couldn't stop thinking about Keefer; the pain was almost unbearable. I never cried so much and for so long. I attempted to stop, and in seconds, I was sobbing again as if my heart were breaking.

The day seemed endless and void of a sunbeam. I wanted to talk to someone, be hugged, and be told this pain would go away. The only person I could think of was a friend that worked at a nearby bank. When I saw her, I broke down and cried again. She came out from behind the desk and gave me a hug, which was wonderful but only helped for the moment. It didn't bring my Keefer back. I wanted to change the hour on the clock and have the day start over. Then Keefer would have stayed in the house forever.

Soon, it would be three forty-five in the afternoon, and Paul would be entering the house. I dreaded the next task at hand, but it had to be done. Telling Paul that his beloved Keefer had passed over the *Rainbow Bridge* was going to crush him.

I was on fire by the time Paul got home from work. I had been crying all day. My eyes showed it, and my head felt it.

Paul came in as usual with a big smile and said, "Everything okay?"

I had trouble getting the words out. I hated to tell him, but I didn't have a choice. When I did, he couldn't believe it. He was sad, angry, mad, and very upset.

He said, "Keefer never went into the road; something must have scared him."

When I told him, I hoped he would take me in his arms and hold me, and we would mourn together. I needed to be held. I was beyond brokenhearted. Paul wanted to see his Keefer. He went to the garage and found him in the plain box the veterinarian had prepared.

We wanted him buried close to us. Paul took him to the edge of the garden. I saw him at the far end of our property, standing so still and holding the box in his hand. Then he dug a very deep hole in our vegetable garden where other animals couldn't find Keefer. He stayed out there for the longest time. I left him alone for his moment with Keefer. He had his own way of mourning and never showed much emotion. This was the only time I ever saw him shed tears.

I was very emotional and cried with very little effort. That was where we were very different. Paul couldn't understand why I cried so easily. I always did, from childhood into adulthood. Losing Keefer was difficult for both of us. I felt as if I cried on and off forever. I couldn't get that awful, sick, lonely feeling to go away. I missed Keefer terribly; I wanted him back. I never mourned to this extent for any human being. That left me feeling guilty. Paul made a cross for Keefer's grave. I ordered a special, custom plaque with his name on it. Our days were dismal for quite sometime. Paul put up a good front. I didn't. I was very sad. I felt as if someone cut a chunk out of my heart.

Every time I cried, I ended up feeling hot all over — especially my head. I did all my usual *things* to cool down, but my emotions kept my body overheated. I lost my appetite; everything tasted like cardboard, but I knew I had to eat something. We had been on such a *happy train ride*, and this incident knocked the wind out of our sails. I didn't know if life was ever going to be the same.

How could I love an animal so much? It was easy to with Keefer.

Finally, the days were a little easier, but not much. I had to keep the thought of Keefer out of my mind. If I didn't, I cried. I wanted another cat to fill Keefer's shoes. That wasn't going to happen. I did find another golden ball of fur looking for a home. We named her Ginger. When Paul came home from work, he wanted to see our new family member. She took off and hid behind the refrigerator. When Ginger finally came out, she ran behind the piano. Eventually, she settled in, but she didn't have Keefer's personality. I actually wanted another Maine coon cat. In 1985, Pepper came to live at the Vona house. When I held Pepper in my arms, I longed for the same feeling I had with Keefer. That didn't happen. I soon realized I needed to stop comparing and enjoy our new additions.

For years, Paul and I had enough trouble taking care of me. Now, it was my responsibility to care of two little ones. This was a positive feature in my healing process. I took over as their mom, and a sensation of maternal love came forth. I didn't have any children of my own, and the cats became my surrogate kids.

Pepper and Ginger were good cats, with their own personalities, and they were enjoyable. They added more life to the house and made us laugh, which was a good characteristic.

In 1986, Paul was working in construction, at a bank in downtown Albany. Unfortunately, he fell and hurt his knee to the extent he couldn't work. Upon returning to work, his union office sent him to another job where they were handling many windows. Often, workmen cut themselves, and nothing comes of it. Some chemical must have been on those windows, because Paul's body erupted with the worst rash I ever saw. He went through all kinds of treatments and drugs, and the rash wouldn't go away. It was so hindering; he had to stop working.

The routine I came to enjoy was drastically altered. Paul understood the bathing and never questioned it, so that wasn't the problem.

Having Paul at the kitchen table, where I did my artwork, took away the quietness I longed for and needed in order to focus. He had too many questions and comments. The atmosphere that is created by a mellow, soft sounding, gentle melody as compared to noisy cars on a racetrack, that was how I was affected mentally. He didn't realize how detrimental it was to my psyche; he was just curious. My freedom vanished. When he was working, I felt unbound and independent.

Without having a hobby of his own, it wasn't long before he was bored and anxious to do something. I tried to block out his comments. "Why are you using that color? Shouldn't it be a different color? Does that look right? How long are you going to draw? When are you getting dressed? When do you think we will leave the house? Aren't you getting a late start?" I was never very good with distractions, and this wasn't any different.

The energy around me changed; it was lifeless and uncreative. I was annoyed. Rushing out the door wasn't my style now. That didn't mesh with the present routine. I began to lose interest but had to pull myself together, or all my dreams would have vanished.

Not long ago, I wanted Paul sitting at the table every morning regardless. I wasn't able to continue without someone being right in the room. Now, I had overcome that fear. I was content to be alone. I didn't want anyone with me. What I really enjoyed was now going to change. I didn't like change, and this new arrangement was stressful.

I couldn't just ignore Paul or leave him home all the time. I loved him; I just wanted my space back.

Finally, our new days together blended and became smoother. After all, it wasn't Paul's fault he was out of work. I just needed to learn how to accept the change and get on with my life.

I stayed with my schedule, and he tagged along. After my morning routine, we usually went to a mall and walked as much as possible. Every day was spent together going someplace.

One gorgeous sunny afternoon in 1987, we went into a local jewelry store. We had shopped there before, but only to look. Paul had known the owner for years. Paul lingered by the ring case and motioned for me to join him. Casually, he told me to pick out a ring. I inhaled too quickly and almost choked. Then I blushed from excitement. The one I finally settled on was, of course, gorgeous. All women probably feel that way. It is a very special moment for all of us.

Paul said if I liked the ring, it was mine. When I was a teen, I had hoped this moment would someday be mine; however, I had doubts. Now, it was real. I received my engagement kiss once we were settled in our car. And along with that, a fuzzy feeling as if soda bubbles were moving throughout my body. Oh, happy days.

We didn't make any arrangements for a wedding at this time.

We had saved a little money, and I asked Paul if a renovation of our kitchen was a possibility. He said yes. I had anticipated this moment for sometime before asking him. My heart rate increased with the excitement of conquering something different. One day, while he was out of the house, I changed into some old clothes. There were empty cardboard boxes in the cellar. I just had to retrieve them. I packed box after box until the kitchen was totally empty, except for the real heavy or permanent items. This was my first time to be all sweaty and get *down and dirty* without looking for air-conditioning. I didn't even think about it. All that was on my mind was to get into something entirely different. Even the heat I felt was acceptable. I wanted to get all the work done before Paul returned home. That way, he would see what I was capable of. I wasn't sure which part was the best: looking forward to the makeover or the fact that I overcame a fear — the fear of leaving my comfort zone to engage in an activity where I might become covered with sweat with no way to cool off.

Finally, this showed me I could and still be okay. Previously, I worked at staying cool all day long. What a relief. Another weight was lifted. I wasn't totally free, but I was getting there. It was the consolation knowing I had ways of cooling myself if necessary. I had air-conditioning when I went to bed and where I ate dinner. And, of course, I started off the day with cool sponge baths.

Paul and his son did most of the renovations. I helped out when asked. As dinnertime approached — and for me that was four o'clock — I changed back into my normal attire and went to an air-conditioned fast food restaurant. Eating there every day wasn't too expensive, because I still brought my own food. I was mainly interested in the temperature and size of the room. A spacious room seemed cooler, which enhanced my appetite. I carried my trusty, canvas, tote bag filled with raw vegetables, a hot vegetable, various fruits, yogurt, and a main course of baked or broiled chicken or meat or fish. I ordered only a diet soda and hot tea, unless it was Pizza Hut. Then I added the salad bar.

The same procedure was followed each day. First, I found the table with cool air moving above the table. Then I ordered a diet soda, took a swallow, and sat there waiting until I was cool enough to eat. A trip to the salad bar disrupted the coolness so, upon returning, I sat a little longer until the cool feeling returned. Next, I proceeded to eat raw vegetables, which were a low-calorie, low-heat food. When I was cold enough, I ate the entree and a hot vegetable. If at any time I felt too warm, a cold, diet soda with ice was on the table. As long as I knew of a way to cool myself down without using cold water, I was fine with eating a considerable amount of *my kind* of food.

I cherished this time of the day. In my dark past, eating was such a chore. Now, I had a cool place to eat, and no one bothered me. I had a few oddities, but overall, I felt this was acceptable progress. I had created a structured day and a time to do each part of it. I didn't see any of it as an obsession. When I compared the present to the dark past, the present day didn't look so bad — not bad at all.

But my migraines were becoming much worse. My neck was stiff, and there was pressure around the right temple. Then the pain shot through my head as if a burning spear was being inserted. I don't know what that actually felt like, but the intensity of the pain was beyond description. Mine never quieted down in a few hours; oh no, they lasted about seventeen hours. It was as if someone were squeezing my brain until it was the size of a pea and then left his or her fist in there. Nothing worked to control the pain. Then I inhaled too much air. This brought about the symptoms of a heart attack. When I felt I couldn't take it anymore, I begged Paul to call 911. The emergency room never helped my migraines, and most of the time, I went home feeling worse than before I went in. There was one good outcome. I was admitted for overnight observation. I was given a drug to knock me out and ease the pain. The next day, my nurse suggested a drug called Fioranal. My doctor prescribed them, and I thought I had found a wonder drug.

Other than the migraines, life was good, even though I continued bathing in cold water every morning. The morning routine of using cold water over and over again on my body worked for me physically and mentally. I wouldn't think of giving it up. At times, the whole *water addiction* was tiring, and it took up too much time, yet I felt I needed it to go on. I convinced myself this was part of my life now, and it was okay.

Paul didn't dare suggest I quit. He learned the *dangerous way* that I wouldn't eat without cold water. And he was right.

My obsessive-compulsive behavior devoured the entire morning, and everything was scheduled around it. I refused doctor appointments, medical tests, and even houseguests. We never left the house early; everything was planned to keep the morning free for my habitual behavior. I wouldn't consider any changes.

One time, Paul said, "What if the house burns down?"

I answered, "It hasn't yet. I'll deal with any situation when it happens. I'm trying to live *in the moment.*"

I never looked toward the bigger picture, only what was in front of me at the time. Now was all that mattered. Perhaps for that reason, I didn't get overwhelmed with my condition. My thinking allowed me to be more positive.

In 1987, the media advocated that people see their doctor for a complete physical with an emphasis on the entire body. I convinced Paul to make an appointment, much to his reluctance. The doctor did many tests, and the results were good. Then Paul's labor union sent him a letter, suggesting he see a lung doctor. Several of the men were getting sick, and it was linked to jobs where asbestos was found. He had a chest X-ray, and we waited for the results.

The follow up appointment was just before his favorite holiday, Christmas. I waited patiently at home with Pepper and Ginger. When he came into the house, he looked as if he had seen a ghost. I asked him what was wrong.

He said, "I have cancer in my lung."

My mouth nearly dropped to the floor. I couldn't believe what I was hearing.

Then he proceeded to tell me what happened on the way home from the doctor's office. He enjoyed going to McDonald's for coffee, and this day was no different. He stopped in, and I am sure he looked rather sad. A gentleman was sitting nearby and asked if he could come over to Paul's table and talk.

He introduced himself. After hearing the news, he asked to pray with Paul. He laid hands on my husband, and Paul said it was a beautiful moment. He told Paul he was a born-again Christian and what church he was affiliated with. He told Paul he had been a very poor man all his life and just made ends meet, but he had always loved the Lord. Then he told Paul he was extremely blessed; he recently won eight million dollars in the New York

State Lottery. Paul and he talked at length about God, church, and faith. Paul found a new friend — one who came along at precisely the right time.

After hearing Paul's story, I was more hopeful than before. We talked more about Paul's new friend than the bad report. His friend told him all about his church, and then Paul said he wanted to go and experience it for himself. He was born a Catholic but hadn't been back to church in years. I was a little more apprehensive due to my childhood experiences, where I learned nothing, and each week I came close to falling asleep during the service. I believed in God and His infinite love, but only through my childhood attendance in church, which conveys how much I didn't learn.

I told Paul I would go with him fairly soon.

For several weeks, Paul attended evening prayer alone. I saw a change in him each time he came home. He was happier and much more positive. I finally joined him for an evening service. The tiny, born-again church was filled with joyfulness and God's love. The music pulled me directly in. I couldn't explain what I was feeling, but it was wonderful. I began singing the words with enthusiasm and excitement. My heart was filled with delight, and I was bursting with gladness. My soul was happy. Now, I knew what Paul was talking about each time he came home from the prayer meetings. I never understood the Bible, and now I wanted to, yet it seemed so overwhelming.

We both went home energized and thirsty for a renewed faith in the Lord. I began talking to God and thanking him for bringing me to Paul and saving me from myself. I prayed for his help and guidance in our journey together and for Paul's healing, which was to rid him of lung cancer. Hope filled my thoughts. There was a possibility to step out of the cold life, and gravitate toward a normal existence of living in a warm temperature zone. I prayed in church, at home, and in my prayer closet over and over and over again.

By the time Paul had his next checkup, the shadow on his lung was gone; the X-ray showed a clean, healthy-looking lung.

We attended church each week. I enjoyed the service, except that I had a difficult time sitting for an hour without getting overheated. I continued to go anyway. Sometimes, the headaches were very bad, and we left early. My doctor prescribed several new migraine medicines; the drugs didn't help. The Fioranal only worked sometimes. I now had temperature changes and migraines to deal with, but it didn't stop me; life was too grand. I seized what I could out of every day. Not until I joined a born-again, Bible-teaching, Christian church did I realize He was with me every step of the way. My faith grew stronger as I continued to walk my walk.

It was now 1988, and we were attending church on most Sundays. Paul adopted my positive outlook, and that made life even better. I believe it was on Paul's mind anyway, but I think something in the Bible prompted him to ask me to marry him. We would become one in God's love; how beautiful was that? I felt as if I were in a dream and didn't want to wake up. I was going to become Mrs. Vona.

Paul decided to read the Bible from cover to cover and in doing so, found the verse that advocates no sex until marriage. I had just discovered great sex and now, no sex? But I knew it was the right thing to do, and that is what we agreed upon. It was a little difficult, but we refrained until after the wedding. It was like going without your favorite dessert for a month, and how wonderful it is when you take pleasure in it once again; only, this was even better.

We didn't want a grand ceremony — just a quiet gathering in our new church with our family and a few friends. Our pastor came to the house for the pre-marriage counseling. Normally, he met with the couple at the church. The pastor knew it would be easier on me in my home. It was nice when someone recognized my suffering with temperature changes.

When I was a little girl, I had visions of a big wedding. My life had definitely changed, and now it was out of the question. Arriving at the church migraine free, and not too warm, was the best I could ask for. And remembering the vows was a little intimidating. Public speaking was always a challenge, and this was no different. I wanted our wedding day to be perfect and special for both of us. I certainly didn't want to let Paul down by forgetting the words.

We decided on an evening wedding at seven. By that hour of the day, my daily routine — I often refer to my obsessive-compulsive behavior as a *routine* because that is how Paul always described it — was about over; and the air was a little cooler, thus, giving us the freedom we needed for the ceremony.

We were married on March 25, 1988; it was a beautiful, balmy seventy degrees. I was a little nervous driving to the church; but when I actually saw the building, then I knew it was real. My knees were trembling, my hands were sweaty, and my heart was racing a mile a minute. It was a good thing I had an arm to hold on to; I don't think I would have made it down the aisle alone. As I stood next to the man I adored, I knew this was the happiest moment of my life. And yes, I remembered the vows.

After a picturesque, evening ceremony and a church filled with smiling faces, we went home and spent the evening together. We knew a reception or honeymoon wasn't possible, and that was fine. I was obsessed with a strict, daily routine. It couldn't be changed even for one night. At home was where

I felt secure and happy, and Paul wouldn't jeopardize that for one day, even if it was our wedding.

What we just experienced was, in itself, completely enough; it was perfect.

I felt bad about Paul missing out on a normal reception or honeymoon, but he said, "As long as I am with you, I don't need anything else."

Looking back to our first days together, I never expected us to be married. He said he loved me right from the first day; it took me a little longer. In those earlier days, my mind was preoccupied with matters of a different nature.

The following day was like any other, back to our routine.

The time set aside for drawing was still in the morning, although now, I experienced a little more activity. There were two cats and a husband to diminish my peace and quiet time.

The migraines were a little more than a bump in the road; however, I continued to draw until they put me to bed. Even without any nutrition, and much time spent in the bathroom, once they passed, I felt renewed. It would have been nice if I could have held on to the renewed feeling. This thought was on my mind after every bad migraine. As soon as I felt good, I busied myself more and more each day; and in about a month's time, I ended up with another migraine. The monthly migraine continued year after year.

Every morning, hot bath and three cold sponge baths — that hadn't changed. And the bath *could not* be any other time of day. I was obsessed with the fact that the bath had to be at this hour, or I was not able to start my day.

About an hour before noon, Paul and I went out for coffee or a diet soda. Dinner routine didn't waver either; I prepared Paul's meal, and he ate at home. Then off we went to Pizza Hut or McDonald's. We continued to sit at the same table every day. Unfortunately, a new heating system was installed, and our spot wasn't always cool; therefore, I brought along a portable, battery-operated, miniature fan. At first, I felt a little conscious using it. Paul heard on the news of an actor carrying a portable fan with him. His was exactly like mine. He was seen using it frequently in restaurants.

Paul said to me, "If JR can use a portable fan, then you shouldn't feel bad about using one. If you need a fan, you just put it right up there on the table, and never mind what people say or think." After that, using the fan didn't worry me. I always placed it on any table, even in the *dress up restaurants*.

Our friends were the employees and the *regulars* of the fast food restaurants. There were brief intervals of conversation where we heard their tales of woe, their joys, the boyfriend/girlfriend problems, and future plans. Paul teased the girls and made them laugh. I shared my art progress. Sounds a little odd; however, that was our world at the time.

After dinner, we walked in a mall or a grocery store. As soon as we returned home from dinner, I put away the perishables from my canvas bag, washed the dishes, did a little exercise to a Richard Simmons record, watched a TV show, and then went to bed. Our daily, predictable schedule didn't change very much.

Chapter 22
Baptized in Water

The church where we were wed started to lean away from what they preached. The members, who were supposedly God's children, began talking about Paul and me. He couldn't take their ongoing, unacceptable whispering, and we were eager to find another church. Paul's new friend and his wife also moved on. The members were interested in his money, and how it could help their church. He directed us to another born-again church outside of Albany. It had a much larger congregation, a wonderful music ministry, great sermons, guest speakers, and various activities.

We attended church almost every Sunday. The songs were different compared to the ones I remembered from years ago. It was a natural thing to do; I lifted my arms to praise and glorify God. In those moments, my body felt perfect; I could feel His presence. I enjoyed the jubilant congregation and their positive outlook. I left, feeling the same way. Hearing God's word and learning more about the Bible was riveting. It was a youthful church, overflowing with love. Life seemed to be very positive for Paul and me.

I continued to pray and ask God for his guidance.

I gave thanks to God for my progress, but I also asked, "Please, no more cold. I want to return to a warm life. It would be nice to enjoy some functions outside my home and interact with people in a warm room."

Little by little, I was getting better. I needed some cold air in my life, but I could tolerate more warmth. I felt as if part of my prayers were being answered.

While attending the previous church, the members talked of an adult baptism. I had never heard of this before. It was to take place in a large tank of water in the church. I was baptized as a baby; however, this was a ceremony for adults. Now, it was his or her choice to accept Jesus as his or her Lord and savior. In doing so, they became born-again in Christ as an adult. I was afraid of the water addiction returning, and I held back on my decision to participate.

In the Bible I was given, Jesus stated that only those who are born again shall see heaven: "Jesus answered him, I assure you, most solemnly I tell you, that unless a person is born again he cannot ever see the kingdom of God." (John 3:3)

The members of our new church were planning the same type of baptism.

Each summer, they held the ceremony at a member's pool, followed by a picnic dinner.

I thought it would be wonderful except for one minor detail: again, the *water*. I had stayed away from swimming for many years. The only time I depended on cold water was in my own warm home after a hot bath. This was a scene from the past: walking into the cool water of a swimming pool. The thought of it made me very nervous and concerned. I wanted to believe it was possible to overcome the fear of going back into the water, especially with my new faith in God becoming stronger. Paul and I never were baptized as adults, and this proclamation before God was very important to us.

Paul and I discussed it at length. Our only concern was my body temperature. The date was set for July. The warm, summer days were in our favor. As the date drew closer, the forecast was hot with plenty of sunshine. This was good news for the water temperature and the air.

I kept saying, "I can do this. I can be baptized in water and not become addicted again. Please, God, help me through this. Please, be with me. I can overcome any fears I once had."

I felt the affirmation was expected of me as a Christian. Besides, now I was a believer; why was I worrying? Even so, I agonized about the one dip in the pool; could I end it there? I told myself I didn't have to swim every day. I could go one time for the baptism, and I'd be fine. I said this over and over and over until I convinced myself it was possible.

It was a hot, summer night, in 1988, and perfect in every way. We drove to the house, parked the car, and walked up near the picnic area. Everyone was happy and very friendly. People were laughing and enjoying the beautiful day. There was a lovely pool right near the house, and my attention was drawn to it as if it were in the center of a stage bathed in bright lights. Once everyone arrived, an announcement was made for the service to begin momentarily.

The church members knew I had an addiction to swimming and cold water, and I hadn't been back in the water in about fifteen years. It wasn't going to be easy, and now was the moment of truth. I was very apprehensive but excited. When it came my turn, I eased myself into the water, and I felt weightless. I was baptized and felt reborn as the water rushed over my head and down my body. It was soothing, comforting, and spiritual — all at the same time. It seemed as if angels were singing all around the pool.

This was an amazing moment. What a long way I had come. I had returned to the water. After the ceremony, I stayed in the water and swam a few laps. When I came out of the pool, I felt refreshed and more alert — temporarily.

I said, "I did it. All thanks be to God."

Paul was baptized next. Soon after the baptism, the food was put on the grill. People were finding a place to sit and eat their dinner. This part was always a little awkward. I only ate at home or in an air-conditioned restaurant — another hurdle I had to overcome someday. For now, the baptism was more than I had hoped for.

As Paul and I were changing our clothes, we discussed the events of the evening. It was especially nice to be at a social gathering with our church friends. Paul said he was extremely proud of me for going into the water. We both thought the members of the church made us feel welcome, and I didn't feel out of place in their company. It was something I wanted more of, if I could get it. I felt that life was coming back in all its glory.

While driving home, I noticed my skin didn't feel the same as it did when we were en route to the baptism. I knew why. I just didn't want to admit it. The answer was the pool water. Not long ago, I was formulating a pile of happy thoughts; yet under it was a little space of doubt, a small chunk of fear, a spot of temptation; and my protective shield was now removed.

I was pleasantly comfortable as we traveled to the event. Now, my skin felt tinged with more heat than was comfortable. I had an instant fear I wouldn't be able to get rid of it. Over the years, I learned to evaluate how my body responded to whatever I put it through. Instantly, I knew what happened. The cool water against my skin caused this unpleasant sensation.

I was content for years without escaping to the pool as my refuge and problem solver. I learned to cope in other ways. By swimming in the water, I stripped away my safeguard. It was as if a gray army of ghosts came back to haunt me.

At this point, the only way to cool myself was to start swimming again. I worked for years to get away from jumping into cold water when I was too hot. I no longer wanted the impulse reaction I once lived with; I was striving toward a time of sufficiently cooling down without anything. Unfortunately, I had thrown myself back into the lake of fire — into temptation.

This scared me, and my one thought was, "What have I done now?"

A pervasive sense of panic set in. Then mumbling to myself in a rationalizing manner, "It's okay. You'll be fine, and tomorrow you will feel just like you did before you went into the pool."

As long as I kept talking to Paul and reminiscing about the party, I was on top of the situation. When I was alone, I was less confident. The gathering was a nice evening out with friends plus positive results for me. The thoughts I carried with me every day were not on my mind: the early morning bathing, carrying my food around, hot and cold temperatures, the eating process, or migraines. All of this vanished for a few wonderful hours; my routine was missing, and I had some freedom.

Now, I questioned my *faith*. Wasn't I strong enough in my beliefs? If I was, then going into the water wouldn't have changed anything. Was the baptism going to satisfy my thirst for swimming, or will I want to try it again? If I did, could I just take a relaxing swim when I wanted to? Was an evil energy waiting, tempting, and just hoping I'd slip?

"Well, enough for today," I said. "I'll just go to bed and see what tomorrow brings."

As Scarlett O'Hara said, "I can't think about that right now. If I do, I'll go crazy. I'll think about that tomorrow."

Chapter 23
Water Addiction Returns

"It's not the load that breaks you down but the way you carry it."
Lena Horn

I had a very peaceful sleep. When I woke, I felt empty. I wanted the day to be the previous night. The baptism had quenched a thirst — filled a hunger spot; I was with God's people and felt so loved. This was a new day, and I had to redirect my thoughts.

Unfortunately, I allowed the brief swim to haunt me. Thoughts bounced around in my brain like balls being blown around in a lottery machine. I weighed the pros and cons of taking up swimming once again. The water had put a spell over me. I convinced myself it wouldn't be like the past. It was more than being too hot this time. I wanted to prove to myself I was getting better and could make these kinds of choices without fear.

Then a voice in my head said, "No, you don't want to go there." The torment — not knowing what to do — continued.

I wasn't sketching in the morning like before. I didn't have the desire. Many of the banks wanted to stop the exhibits. Sales were dwindling; so to move my stock of artwork, I dropped the price on all paintings to five dollars. I thought the paintings would fly off the wall. We sold a few; however, I felt it was a sign to either change or stop drawing.

The days were long and nonproductive. I was restless. By now, my hair was down to my waist and quite warm and very annoying. I had this wild desire to cut it all off, shorter hair seemed to be the answer.

I was playing games with myself. The haircut was only a temporary relief from the heat. In truth, I had decided to take up swimming once again.

This was a huge makeover, a monumental change. The thought of surprising Paul was also a fun idea. Before I changed my mind, I took off for the closest mall in search of a hair salon.

I wanted my hair extremely short. Once I started swimming, a wet head with long hair would be a nuisance, plus it would lower my body temperature when I was in air conditioning.

I said to the hairstylist, "Cut it ALL off. Not just a trim, I want it cut short, leave about an inch all over my head."

The hairstylist did as I said. I felt better than my hair looked. There was nothing there. It even was odd to touch, as if I had peach fuzz all over my head. I was pleased with the new me. It was a bit drastic; however, I had been desperate for something very new. I was free of hairdressers, appointments, and finding someone able to do tight braids. Plus the hair wasn't restricted anymore, and possibly, it would grow back on the right side of my head.

I returned home with a bounce in my step and a big smile. I looked straight at Paul and waited for his reaction. He didn't say much: it took some getting used to; he liked it, if I liked it. I expected more than that.

The excitement of a new hairdo faded quickly when it came time to eat lunch. I was hoping the haircut would make that easier. I must have thought the haircut gave me special powers to lessen the heat. Without lying down to cool off, I attempted to have a bite to eat. Every place in the house felt too warm. I opted for the garage where I opened a door. It was too warm there as well, and I ate very little. This wasn't good. I felt trapped in heat once again. I was banking on the idea of a new haircut, but it let me down.

I needed a routine for the upcoming days. I wasn't going to suffer every day as I once did because I couldn't cool myself enough to eat. The past wasn't going to happen all over again. I didn't want to end up in the hospital. Fear began to take over. I didn't see a light at the end of a tunnel or a solution for eating at home. I finally came up with a hopeful plan. My only other option was a restaurant. I said not a word to Paul. Negative energy would have interfered with my strategy. Instead, I talked to myself, which was probably worse.

Whenever I allowed my mind to consider a change, unfortunately, I was reminded of where I could and could not exist. Putting up a barrier only stopped advancement. I knew this to be true, yet fear was a rather strong factor in the equation.

On this day, I tried to delete all of that thinking. I only thought about my goal. The house was becoming too warm, and I was having difficulty eating my meals. On the other hand, my lifestyle would be altered. Fear was still prohibiting a decision. The following thoughts had to be dealt with in order for this venture to be successful:

First — leave the secure nest.
Second — cope with traffic, which might hold up breakfast. The last time I waited in traffic before breakfast was when I was on my way to the swimming pool in the seventies. This was very different.
Third — dine with strangers at breakfast. Paul was the only one I saw at home. We made sure it stayed that way. We didn't want any interference with

the daily bathing ritual or meals.

Fourth — no sponge bathing in cool water before breakfast.

Fifth — dress in street clothes at breakfast. Every day for ten years, since 1978, I had worn sleepwear to breakfast at Paul's house. There is nothing wrong with that, except I refused to dress differently. Apparently, a few of my obsessions were going to be turned upside down.

While lying in bed that evening, again I addressed the heat dilemma. I had decided what to do. It would begin the next day. If every part of the plan was secure in my mind, then maybe I could pull it off. This involved getting out of bed, taking a shower, getting dressed, putting a few food items in my canvas bag, and then driving to McDonald's for breakfast. I never would have thought of doing this a month ago. I prayed for success. I asked God to help me overcome my fears. Standing strong on my thoughts, I believed in myself.

I didn't think of the obstacles along the way, only the prize at the end. My confidence was strengthened by repeating the positive steps from the beginning of the day until I walked through the restaurant door. I left out all possible doubts. This new challenge had to work. When a situation comes down to *no other option*, as a rule, I succeed and move forward.

I assumed very few cars would be on the road early in the morning. As it turned out, everyone must have been going to work when I was on my way to McDonald's. If that wasn't bad enough, the cars were backed up at the traffic light. Before leaving the house, I took a very cool shower. It was useless as I sat in the hot car, waiting for the light to change. Waiting and watching, my heart rate increased. I gripped the steering wheel harder and bit my lip, as if that would help. If only the light would change. I was sure it was stuck. The anxiety lessened as I did some deep breathing exercises and tried to focus on what I was about to do. I finally made it to the parking lot.

In our home, the temperature was fairly consistent. This is what I was accustomed to. I needed an even temperature in order to keep the migraines under control, keep the body temperature where it belonged, and to function properly. Once I walked out the door, I was no longer in charge. A restaurant could be very inconsistent, possibly different each day. And most likely, I'd have to wait in line. I knew it was imperative to concentrate on the whole picture and what I was trying to accomplish. I had to *stay in the moment* and not let my fears get the best of me.

Try to put yourself in the following scene and count all the temperature changes: lift the bed covers away from your body; shower; put on clothes; move to the outdoors; sit inside your car; exit the car into the weather of the particular day; walk inside a restaurant to the dining area; and, *if nature calls*, occupy the restroom.

Then there is the trip home. In all, that could be more than eleven varying temperature changes. My body doesn't have time to adjust to any of them before I am thrown into the next one. This was quite a challenge. Over the years, I conditioned myself to a controlled environment inside our home. I put myself into my own *protected bubble*. Now, I was going to venture out of that element and enter into an unknown area. I had no control over the environment around me.

Once I arrived at the restaurant, the first day worked beautifully. It was exciting. Breakfast tasted divine, and I adjusted perfectly. The temperature at McDonald's wasn't cold, just a little cooler than outside. I was anxious to tell Paul what I accomplished. He couldn't believe I ate breakfast someplace other than home. He was happy I initiated such a drastic move. We both accepted my venture as progress. After the initial excitement wore off, I felt empty and useless; there was no purpose to the day.

I heard myself saying, "Now what do I do?"

The house still felt too warm, and I was very uneasy. I decided to call a friend. She and her husband stood up for us at our wedding. They both loved the Lord, and when I was around either of them, I felt all was right with the world. The couple had a beautiful, new pool and told us the welcome mat was always out. I was sure I wouldn't be going into the water; I didn't want to be tempted.

My friend was easy to be around, always smiling and laughing. Several times, she invited me to come over for a swim. I thought it best to resist, yet something kept telling me to say yes.

After about a week of McDonald's and interacting with people, I longed for companionship other than Paul. And while doing the household chores, I was becoming warmer and warmer. I was tired of fighting the heat monster. Subconsciously, I was being led back to cool water. The desire became too strong, and I was too weak. I longed for the water; I was vulnerable, so why not enjoy it? I finally gave in.

During the summer of 1988, I went swimming three times every day, took a warm shower twice a day, and one cool shower per day.

The water eased all tension, and my body was totally relaxed. My friend encouraged me to swim in the pool anytime. I enjoyed being back in the water, and this time, the water was tepid. I wasn't freezing myself. The only problem was her house had central air. This could become a danger zone as I passed through the cold on my way to the dressing room. I always brought along a digital thermometer to check my body temperature. If I turned white or didn't feel well, it was time to take a reading.

Not long after I returned home, I was anxious to get back to the pool. Together, the sun and the water made up the perfect pill for feeling healthy and alive. Swimming put a spark in each day. The cool water was instant; whereas, waiting for my body to cool on its own took a long time. I was getting a great tan and some very good exercise. The decision of what to do with the day was no longer a problem. I had a new destination, but there was a down side. I was being drawn to the pool as if it were a magnet. I didn't see where this was heading.

I felt I was becoming a nuisance and taking advantage of my good friend. Not far from her house was a hotel with an indoor and outdoor pool. I talked to Paul about a membership, and we agreed I should purchase one. I also checked out our town pool. It was about ten minutes from our front door, and a summer pass was very inexpensive. I ended up with two new places to swim.

Before I knew it, the whole day was taken up with swimming, driving, and eating. I didn't even realize the familiar pattern.

Every day, I was eating three meals at McDonald's and still lugging food around in a huge, canvas bag. I had been obsessed with a daily ritual at home. When I took off for the fast food restaurant, I was happy to break away from the pattern. My routine at McDonald's appeared more normal because I was out in public, pretending to be different than the person I was at home. It seemed less obvious. I was far from normal, because I was obsessed with doing the same thing every day. The only difference was I was doing my *thing* outside my home instead of inside my home. Danger wasn't far away, and I was too blind to see it.

I was free to do as I pleased all day long; nevertheless, I felt guilty every morning as I left the house at sunup. I believe that was why I made my secretive exit quiet and quick. If I was okay with what I was doing, I probably would have kissed Paul and left with a smile on my face. Instead, I was nervous and anxious. I had let go of some obsessions. Regrettably, this new lifestyle was still an obsessive-compulsive behavior, and it was more dangerous.

As each day dawned, I felt the *haunting past* begin to creep up on me. I swiftly focused on my needs at the moment and not the frightening outcome. Here I was once again, taking up the entire day with eating and swimming. Plus, the uneasy warm feeling I used to encounter at daybreak was returning. To ease the tension and become more undisturbed, I increased the migraine drug Fioranal. It lessened the stress. I was able to cope with the insane schedule I had created.

I took one pill while sitting in bed and waited for my body to become calm, cool, and collected. Next, the usual routine of a shower, put on some clothes, pack up the food, and leave the house. None of that changed. Anything needed for breakfast was always prepared the evening before to save time, so I wouldn't overheat.

Each morning at breakfast, when the repetitive behavior was over, I gave a deep sigh of relief. I admitted to myself that swimming was easier than my other daily ordeal. But progress isn't supposed to be uncomplicated. Most every morning, I headed back home feeling rather pumped. I relayed to Paul all that occurred from the time I left in the morning. A small fraction of this new experience was a step forward in my healing; and it was beneficial. At the time, my thinking wasn't quite as clear. I only saw what I wanted to see.

I was barely home an hour before I was on my way out the door again. I put together another canvas bag — which held my bathing suit, towel, and suntan lotion — and quickly headed to the hotel pool. The buzz throughout the hotel was exciting, and the people were friendly. The sun was shining and the pool was gorgeous. It was heaven on Earth.

I changed into my bathing suit and eagerly walked out into the sun — yes, the sun. I prayed to God every day that I would become a normal person, one who could tolerate the heat. Little by little, I was taking pleasure in the warmth of the rays. However, I still needed a cool swim. And when it was mealtime, I chose a moderately cool environment plus a little cool air above my head.

I saw a transformation taking place. I was able to enjoy a considerable amount of warmth *outdoors and indoors, which* was rather amazing, considering where I had come from. I hadn't reached the point of eating in a warm environment. That would happen when it was time.

When I swam years ago, I concentrated on the swimming only. This time around, I didn't feel like an addict. I was lying in the sun, socializing occasionally, swimming, and being part of the summer scene.

My skin was more exposed than it had been in years. It felt strange not having by body mostly covered. Out of the sun, I chilled very easily. It made me want to curl up in a fetus position and hold in what little heat I produced. Therefore, I was eager to lie in the sun and feel its warmth soak into my bones. I lasted much longer than I anticipated. In fact, I lay there until I couldn't take the heat any longer; it felt that good. I was, in fact, out in the sun. That concept gave me warm, fuzzy goose bumps. This was certainly progress. This scene was possible because of the pool. If cool water was all I needed, then a cold shower should suffice. Not so. There was something about first lying still and allowing the heat to build up in my body. Next, I was convinced a cool swim was the only way to adjust the abundance of heat I felt. I had concocted a formula. When both elements were complete and my brain was satisfied, then I could please my stomach with a meal. After many years of thriving in the cold, I didn't think the sun would ever feel good.

I preferred to be at McDonald's before the noon rush. I didn't take pleasure in long lines; it only heated me up. I was more interested in finding a table where I could sit and cool down before I ate. I took another pill, ate my lunch, and then drove back to the pool. At around two o'clock, I left the hotel and returned home.

It wasn't long before I was back in the car and on my way to the town pool for more of the beautiful sunshine and cool water. When I arrived at the pool, I never entered the water immediately. I had to lay in the hot sun first, and then only when my body was extremely warm did I enter the pool.

If the day was cloudy, I looked to the heavens and searched for a patch of blue or a glimpse of the sun. It had to be up there somewhere. Then I became mad at the weatherman for not giving me a sunny, hot day. How could I eat without my set pattern, the formula? The water wasn't inviting on cloudy days, but I wouldn't allow myself to depart without taking a swim first. When the air temperature read ninety, I was in my glory. Most people were complaining of the horrific heat, but I was lovin' it. I never thought for one minute my lips would speak those words.

After a few laps in the pool, I returned home where I showered and dressed for dinner. In between all of this, I briefly talked to Paul. Sadly, my interests were outside our home. For the last meal of the day, I returned to McDonald's with my canvas bag filled of food.

I was on a ride going nowhere, being eaten up by an obsession.

At first, the swimming was exciting; however, after three months of swimming at one pool or another, it was becoming a chore, as was the driving to each destination. Many days, I was so tired and didn't want to do any of it. In order for me to continue this craziness and to diminish the migraines, I increased the Fioranal medicine. One pill wasn't strong enough. I took one at daybreak and two pills at each meal, totaling seven pills each day. Now, I was not only addicted to the swimming/sun routine but the pills as well, and I wasn't able to stop.

Paul thought I was just plain enjoying myself, so he never interfered. Plus he didn't see me all that much. It was difficult for him to evaluate my wacky schedule. Even if Paul tried to warn me in a pleasant manner, I was very convincing at stating my case to anyone.

One day, I ran into my good friend. She was the gal with the beautiful pool, where I first started swimming. On this particular day, she was at the hotel swimming pool.

Leaving normal behind and entering the addictive stage changed my persona. My obsessive-compulsive behavior took on a consistent schedule, leaving very little time to socialize. I preferred not to talk; it hindered the process. I heated up in the sun and then quickly swam in the cool pool. Conversation after a swim only detained me, which, in turn, allowed the heat to creep back into my body, thus, interfered with lunch. I didn't foresee meeting anyone I knew at the hotel. When I did, the result was embarrassing.

Our meeting was brief and rather cold. This not how she remembered me. When my friend saw me away from the pool, I was an entirely different person, overflowing with conversation and warmth. I soon learned how this addiction pulled me away from the people I loved — and who loved me.

The swimming was something I wanted to enjoy on my own, but I think it went further than that. I was being very secretive. Interacting with strangers was fine; however, I didn't want to bump into anyone who I recognized. The truth be known, I didn't want Paul to see or be with me at the pool either. I would gladly talk about my day later on. That way, he wasn't observing my ritual or the shocking realization I was reliving a part of my dark past. With that kind of thinking, I should have known my behavior was wrong. There was no shame in going swimming. The *daily, obsessive behavior* was the damaging element.

Deep down, I think I knew where I was headed because a similar scene played out years ago. This time, I had my faculties, but I was still addicted. As I left the pool, I knew I was slipping backward. Before long, the food didn't satisfy my taste buds, and I was constantly too warm. Swimming, showering, or air-conditioning wasn't correcting the problem. The summer was ending, and each day became a struggle. It was not fun anymore.

"Oh, my God, what am I doing?" I said. "This can't be happening again."

Even so, I continued my obsessive behavior.

The summer of 1988 was coming to an end. The seasons were changing. The days were cooling down. The sun wasn't as hot; the pool was not as appealing. The hot days increased my urgency and desire to swim, whereas the chilly weather had just the opposite effect. Even so, I found it impossible to stop that gnawing pain of wanting it. There was an energy pulling me in — a force I couldn't resist. I was allowing myself to be drawn back into the water. I was addicted again. I didn't need the extreme cold, but it was the combination of both the sun and the water. The thrill was wonderful for the first month. I continued because I allowed my brain and body to follow the craving. I knew I had to end this facade, but how?

Every time I visited the pool, I argued with myself. The weather was too cool, or the pool temperature was too warm, or the sun wasn't shining. The enjoyment was gone.

The day was like any other day except it was the end of September, and it was gloomy and cool and spitting droplets of water from above. I had a migraine even though I was taking all the headache pills. I parked the car. I didn't feel like moving. It seemed as if I sat there forever, watching people pass by my car. They looked my way and smiled. Then I watched as their bodies moved toward the nice, warm building. On previous days, I witnessed this same scene. I knew they were about to ease themselves into the indoor pool and comment on how comfortable the water temperature was — *warm*. Oh, how I wanted to be like them. It would alleviate tremendous stress and pain if I could endure any kind of temperature without becoming ill.

An inner voice was telling me not to swim. I refrained from stepping out of the car into the damp, cold rain. I told myself, "In a minute; I'll move in a minute or two." If I couldn't swim in cold water, how would I eat dinner? Yet the thought of food made me nauseous. I didn't feel well at all. The whole summer had been a grueling pace. I was exhausted. I believed the best idea was to turn the car around and go home. My head was pounding to the extent my eyes hurt. I wasn't sure I could make it home. I took a couple of deep breaths, started the car, and moved forward. All I could think about was getting into bed.

As soon as I returned home, I took my body temperature. I stood waiting for the digital beep to stop; the reading was a low ninety degrees. I felt sick to my stomach as I ran to the bathroom to vomit. The sleepless night seemed to go on forever. Agonizing pain pressed down upon my entire head. I felt as if it might rip apart. With each trip to the toilet, I prayed I was closer to the end of the migraine. I thrashed around in my bed, looking to find some relief, but the pounding in my forehead and temples continued through the night. My head felt as if someone was cutting it in half and taking his or her time at it.

Chapter 24
How Does Your Garden Grow?

I survived into the next day; we generally do. I thought the pain would never end, but it did. The only things I obtained from the summer were a good tan and plenty of exercise.

The day looked brighter than yesterday. I was surprisingly relieved the swimming had stopped. For now, my tired body wasn't going anywhere. Paul fixed me a beautiful poached egg on toast, accompanied with green tea. It tasted marvelous. When lunch rolled around, I was too nervous and afraid to eat solid food. Once again, I had taken a big step backward where I depended upon the cool water prior to eating.

My routine was dismantled. But not to worry, I'd have a new one shortly. In the meantime, I prepared a cup of bouillon and drank a Coke. Mentally, I chose to believe in these two items. I proclaimed them *safe*. I obtained enough temporary warmth from the bouillon to keep my body temperature up. The cold drink, on the other hand, made me *feel* cool but was really creating body heat through the sugar in the drink. I assumed the two would balance each other. I was uncertain about the reaction of any solid food; therefore, I allowed my brain to only accept the consumption of Coke and bouillon when I didn't have cool water as a device in which to cool my body. At least for the moment, I wouldn't overheat, and my body temperature would stabilize.

The day was uneventful but relaxing. My whole body said, "Cool it," and that is exactly what I did.

When it was time for dinner, I suggested we go to a different McDonald's rather than the one I was going to daily. This was a good way to start changing the order of things. Again, I brought what I needed in my canvas satchel; some things took longer than others to change. The indoor temperature was perfect, and everything I ate tasted fantastic. I walked outdoors after dinner just to breathe life back in. I couldn't get enough of the mild, warm air as it brushed against my face. It was September, and yet that last little bit of soft, summer air was lingering about, as if God saved it for me to enjoy just before He opened a door to let in the long, cold winter. The fast pace ended, and I felt calm. I wanted to stand in the parking lot with my eyes shut and feel and smell the air forever. The swimming episode was finished. Instead, I was enjoying a beautiful, late afternoon with my husband. In exchange for the swimming, I was given this ideal moment. Life was back on track.

Upon leaving the restaurant, I desperately wanted another day just like this one. Regrettably, the next day was cooler. I went to the same restaurant. The inside was a different temperature from the day before. I know two days can never be exactly the same. I had just vowed to change the order of things, and here I was, trying endlessly to accomplish the impossible. I became terribly upset and agitated because the room wasn't the same. I desperately wanted the previous day back. I was finding happiness on perfect days; I desired more of them.

I was somewhat sure swimming could no longer be a part of my life. Once again, I had allowed the addiction to pull me downward into a dark hole. It appeared one swim wasn't going to cut it. I thought I had enough faith in God, and my willpower was strong. Evidently, I wasn't ready. There was more work to be done. I had to grow in other ways. When the time was right, I would succeed.

Every time I crash, something good comes out of it. I shed one more negative layer — a layer that hopefully falls away from my life forever. And with this last crash, all of the headache pills ended. I wanted a clean, fresh slate — no prescription drug dependencies. Second, the search for coolness was over. I had made a complete turnaround. I enjoyed being out in the sun. Even a warm, summer breeze was acceptable. There were some unusual changes.

Once the swimming stopped, I couldn't tolerate a windy day. A warm, gentle breeze was all right for a brief moment, as long as I had a hat on my head; anything longer produced a headache or a migraine. If the air was on the cool side, my body temperature dropped. I suppose some of those things don't qualify as a positive outcome; however, moving forward and away from anything cold sounded like progress. The life Paul and I lived for many years was about to make a drastic transformation. We used to look for cold or cool; now, we needed a warm environment with no moving air. This extreme change was difficult to believe. It was so different compared to searching for cold temperatures. I didn't need a fan or cold air blowing down on my body. How many long years had I nourished this idea? And now, it was delivered. I was finally content to sit and enjoy the natural stillness around me. It was divine. This was a huge lifestyle change. I had prayed for it constantly. I didn't want to live in cold anymore. And here it was being handed to me. I didn't give up anything when I stopped swimming. I gained a great deal of comfort for myself and for others. I looked forward to visiting my friends and relatives without a desperate urge to flee into the cold.

The obsession to use water as a tool was becoming less. I had to pinch myself to make sure it was I, Jill. I was, in fact, right here in the middle of this beautiful awakening and newfound freedom.

I need patience when waiting for God — another lesson.

The swimming stopped; dining at McDonald's three times a day continued.

The winter came and went, and I became stronger with each passing day.

I always drove by the same houses on my way home, but on this spring day in 1989, I seemed to be more observant than the year before. One house, in particular, caught my eye. There was a multitude of beautiful flowers everywhere. I had never seen so many hosta plants in one area. Something in my soul told me to stop and take a look. The woman of the house was in her garden. She barely acknowledged me standing there as she busied herself in this paradise. A soda in one hand and a cigarette burning in the ashtray gave me the feeling this passionate gardener enjoyed these two things as much as her flowers. Her garden must have taken up a lot of her time because there wasn't a weed in sight.

I complimented her on her gorgeous sanctuary; it was so calm and peaceful and meticulously neat. She was a bit preoccupied with what she was doing. I wasn't sure if I was bothering her; nevertheless, she took the time to answer my long list of horticultural questions.

As I listened to this avid gardener, my mind was already planning a similar landscape. Before I stepped back into my car, I knew what I wanted, and that was to have lots of my own flowers everywhere.

Paul and I always planted a few annuals every spring. He always worked the soil and then planted the flowers. I watched, because I was afraid of becoming too warm with no way to cool off. After visiting this fine, hardworking lady, I wanted to be involved. I never did any gardening in the past.

My grandmother was very active in the garden club and won all kinds of ribbons on her ability to arrange flowers. She had gorgeous flowers all around her house. I always admired my grandparents for their hard work. It certainly paid off; the colors and array of flowers were magnificent.

When I was younger, the thought of working in the soil and becoming sweaty wasn't appealing. On this particular day, I was ready to get started. I began to think outside my safe, secure box. I wanted to move to a new level in my healing. Deep down in my heart, I knew I could do the work. The time was right; I was right for the time. It was a new challenge. I would rise above it and make it happen.

I couldn't get home fast enough to share my excitement with Paul. He was also eager and ready to start our project. Covering our property with flowers required some thinking and planning before we even picked up a shovel. The local nurseries supplied us with wonderful information. Paul wanted to please me, and, in turn, that made him happy. He saw I was growing and spreading my wings. He believed his purpose in life was unfolding. Paul was beginning to see his independent woman.

Each challenge I tackled was a big improvement from what he saw in 1978: a thin girl in her thirties, frail and underweight with extreme low body temperature, very vulnerable, and didn't know what was happening to her body.

Many times over the years, Paul said, "I want you to get as healthy, as strong, and as independent as you possibly can while I am still alive."

When Paul saw me taking charge and advocating such a big undertaking, he knew I was growing toward a better tomorrow. Then Paul came up with a very unusual suggestion.

He said, "Okay, this is my idea. We want a drastic change in our yard. We want to eliminate mowing grass. What do you think about adding mounds of dirt sporadically all over the property, front and back? Then cover everything with mulch and plant your flowers?"

I liked it; it sounded creative and unusual with some character. This layout would be different from any other property. We had the most horrible grass of any yard on the street. Possibly, a nice landscape was about to happen. I was eager yet overwhelmed; both emotions came over me at the same time. This was going to be an enormous project. At the same time, I felt it would be something I'd appreciate forever.

The mulch was delivered and deposited in the street. Half of the load needed to be in the front garden; the other half brought to the back garden. Paul was enthusiastic and full of energy. He filled his wheelbarrow full of mulch and started to whittle away at the massive pile. After awhile, I stopped counting the trips; I believe there were eleven yards to be distributed. Each afternoon, I spent about an hour working in our garden. Paul did all the heavy labor, including the planting of the shrubs. My job entailed doing the layout, planting all the perennials, fertilizing everything, and then thoroughly watering every plant. Our masterpiece began to take shape.

Little by little, our garden was coming together. Not all of the neighbors were as positive as we were. The look was imaginative and out of the ordinary. Our house was always a little different; why change character now?

Paul once told me, "I don't care about the outside world; here is all that matters."

Chapter 25
Determination

It is no longer crucial for me to live in a *refrigerator*. As I look back in time, it makes me shiver.

I made it a practice to evaluate how my body reacted to varying temperatures. Over the years, I put myself through many extreme changes. I was determined to acquire the environment I needed at the time. My new life was just the opposite of how I once lived. The thing was, Paul and I had a difficult time finding warm temperatures with no moving air. And every year thereafter, it wasn't much different. Therefore, the freedom was not what I anticipated.

I found my new *comfort-healing zone* needed to be warm. Everything in my body worked better. I called it BBB — brain, bowel, and body temperature. All three were severely screwed up in the cold zone.

My goal was to become a warm human being who *enjoyed* being warm. In order to reach such a point, it required God's help, and I had to do my part as well.

I learned food choice is imperative in determining comfort or discomfort. It was important to eat a wholesome, balanced diet and include good fats and natural sugars. To add heat in the diet, I included olive oil, avocados, walnuts or cashews, pasta and potatoes, and rice. These foods aided in the elevation of my body temperature. I kept my body cool with plenty of the following fruits: cantaloupe, honeydew, blueberries, peaches, nectarines, grapes, and apples.

Some fruits created more heat, such as bananas, watermelon, mango, and pears. They were used more sparingly or when I needed to boost the numbers on the thermometer. Most vegetables were fine. I found carrots and raw mushrooms to be my favorite. I ate so many carrots my fingers turned a yellowish orange color. It almost looked as if I had jaundice. Fat-free yogurt and lots of water was a nice way to finish a meal. These foods also helped to level off any heat build up.

I don't eat much meat, although, occasionally, if I feel chilled, lack energy, have low body temperature, and I crave something, but I don't know what it is, I will splurge and eat a Whopper or a Big Mac.

In the past, when I ate one of these, my whole body felt as if it were engulfed in heat. I had to be in motion constantly. Sitting in one place was almost unbearable. Consequently, I feared eating such foods. If I gave in and indulged, I disliked myself intensely. The suffering was so unpleasant; I should have known better. Yet they tasted so good. I envied people who could eat anything they wanted and not be affected by too much body heat.

I am proud to say that finally, I can tolerate one of those delicious burgers occasionally. After the first bite, I smile. Then I close my eyes while I delight in every morsel. Foods play a large role in stabilizing my body temperature. Warm surroundings are just as important. That doesn't mean living in Florida or in a hot environment. It means a warm, comfortable home throughout the day, a warm car, warm commercial buildings, and no moving air at anytime. Also, on a windy day, in any season, my body temperature generally drops.

I know what I should do in order to maintain this *safety zone*, which keeps me away from the hospital. But sometimes I break out of *the bubble* and indulge anyway. I am thirsty for life, experiences, and memories. Sometimes, it works out; other times, I pay the consequences.

Our home is about the only place where I am able to sustain the temperature I require. But I am determined to beat the odds. I will persist in battling the outside world until it, too, becomes a comfortable spot for me to exist, when I so choose.

I continued to see Dr. Howard, at least, two to four times a year. She often drew several vials of blood. It was part of the routine checkup. My weight was documented upon each visit. I was weighed facing away from the scale numbers. I didn't see the point; I was well past that part of my life. The attending nurse said this was the new protocol for most patients afflicted with eating disorders — past or present. Each time, when I asked what my weight was, I received an answer, which was good enough for me.

My doctor listened and documented my complaints and improvements. She was always interested in what was going on in my life, how the artwork was progressing, if Paul was okay, and things, in general. Dr. Howard had great bedside manner. She took a sincere interest in all phases of my life; a note of progress or regression was always made in my life. She was always on the lookout for a miracle pill for the migraines and my discomfort with environmental temperature changes and relayed any findings to me. I filled many prescriptions but didn't take any one drug very long. We had a standard joke between us on the subject. She knew me so well by now. Most of the time, it was useless to suggest any drug; however, one never knows, and at least, she made a strong effort. I suffered enough in my life. If a drug intensified the suffering, I discontinued taking a pill when it added misery to my day.

My prayers were answered. I didn't have the need to be cold. I was finally in the warm sector of my life. Many buildings were being renovated at the same time. Who would have thought the owners would install new heating systems with cool, moving air? Not I. The timing wasn't in our favor; that was for sure.

At the point in my life when I didn't require a cold flow of air, that's exactly what I found in most restaurants, and all my meals became very stressful. I never knew what I would find when I arrived at an eatery. There were several restaurants I frequented. When one wasn't suitable, I moved on to the next. I never gave up trying to find the perfect temperature. When I did, I was able to consume a meal. Not once did I return home. I drove from restaurant to restaurant until one was acceptable.

One of my favorite restaurants became extremely cold. People continued to sit in the dining area with their coats on. When anyone asked for heat, the manager ignored the request. I never figured it out; maybe I wasn't supposed to. A few times, I made the attempt to eat my dinner in the cold; however, along with suffering, either my body temperature dropped, I acquired a migraine headache, or both.

Another fast food chain decided to renovate part of their building. The entire main dining room was temporarily inaccessible. The table I sat at every day was unavailable. One way or another, I didn't give up eating at this restaurant. The only room open for business was called the atrium. It had a lot of windows, which made it very chilly. If I sat at one particular table, then I was able to feel some warm air trickle in from the inaccessible room. I desperately wanted this table every day.

I was afraid to look toward my favorite table and find someone sitting there. When I was lucky, the table was mine. As I settled into my seat, I let out a deep sigh of relief. Each day, I went through the same stressful fear.

Normally, winter is frigid. The atrium was made up of almost all windows. The sun left the room early at this time of the year, making the room unpleasantly cold. The dining area was way too cool; my stubbornness kept me there. I convinced myself it was too much work to find another eatery, and most likely, it wouldn't have been any better. I wanted to be in charge of the heating system, so to satisfy my unsettling spirit, I hung on to the hope of someone turning up the heat. Through my controlling personality, I complained and almost begged the manager to comply. Unfortunately, the room didn't become any warmer. The food I consumed didn't put enough fuel in my body.

Cold air and no heat in my body only added up to one thing: a drop in my core temperature. When I looked down at my hands, they were turning white. I immediately knew it was Raynaud's syndrome. It was difficult to move them, and the pain radiated throughout all the fingers. I continued to sit there. Getting some nutrition was more important. The same incident happened on and off in previous years. I was on a restricted diet, and I drank low-calorie soda with ice. I also sat too long in very cool temperatures. The result was white, unhealthy-looking fingers.

My understanding is the blood vessels constrict when the body is cold in order to keep the inner core warm. If the body continues to lose heat, then the brain is in trouble. The brain is top priority. The body will sacrifice blood when it's cold, so there is enough for the brain. The other odd thing is your hands will feel cold when they are losing heat; your head won't. When the blood departs from the fingers, it is also very painful.

I quickly finished eating and went to my car. As soon as I sat myself down, I turned the car heater up to the highest level. I quickly grabbed the digital thermometer from the glove compartment and took a reading of my body temperature. It read ninety-two degrees. That only meant one thing: go straight home and warm up. The first thing I did when I arrived home was to slip into bed. Then I quickly pulled all the covers up over my head and escaped into *revival land*. This traps the heat. Taking in long, deep breaths and exhaling slowly, I waited for my body temperature to rise. Normally, a bad headache accompanied being too cold. As the migraine started to disappear, I knew my body core was warming. I began to feel much better only because my body temperature was close to normal.

Sometimes, I was just too chilled, and I needed Paul's extra body heat. I often asked him to join me in bed and hold me close. In a matter of minutes, I could feel the heat accumulating throughout my entire body. His body was always extremely warm, and doing this quickly raised my temperature. After about five minutes, the thermometer read ninety-eight point six degrees.

Even with all the pain, I was persistent in putting myself through this obsessive-compulsive behavior every day. Each time I arrived home, I complained to Paul about the conditions. It never served any purpose, except I was able to vent my feelings. He patiently listened; what else could he do?

When my body couldn't take the torture anymore, ironically, a migraine developed. This was probably a sign telling me to take a breather; my body needed some *downtime*. The only way to rid myself of the intense pain was bed rest. The following day, I had my usual Coke and hot beef bouillon.

When I was housebound, I ate as little food as possible, only enough for some energy and body heat. I was persistent in keeping the same thoughts about consuming solid food. It was two simple equations: eat solid food and need a large open area to walk; or eat light liquids and be temporarily content to stay in the house. By the third day, I returned to the same fast food restaurant where I continued to struggle with the elements and complained of the cold.

I was driven in one direction or another. In the past, I had to swim in order to eat. Now, I was leaving my home on a daily basis and eating three meals at a fast food restaurant because I couldn't bring myself to eat at home. Even though both obsessions were created to deal with the heat I felt, I put myself though an exhausting behavior that nearly defeated me.

There were mornings when I didn't want to take a bath before I left the house or to leave the house at all. Thoughts raced around in my head constantly. If I didn't bathe, I was afraid I couldn't eat once I got to the restaurant; therefore, I had to continue my obsession each day. I vowed not to eat at home. One way or another, this repetitive behavior would work. The problem was I was fixated with continuing the pattern even when I didn't want to do it.

After awhile, I believe my body retaliated; it wanted to hang around for a while longer. Paul suggested trying another location of the same chain restaurant. I procrastinated about switching. I wasn't big on change, but I finally gave in. The first day I went to the other store, they were very busy, and the lines were long. By the time I received my food and sat down, I was too warm to eat much of anything. A senior citizen was working there at the time. She was kind and understanding and appeared to recognize some of my problems. When she saw me all flustered and very uneasy, she knew I needed some help.

The kind senior said, "Go take a table; write down what you want. I'll get it for you and bring it to the table."

This older gal was a real sweetheart and made life a little easier. She sensed my pain and anguish and came to my aid.

In the winter, the road conditions were often hazardous. Whatever the weather was, I was determined to go out of the house for breakfast, lunch, and dinner. The most difficult time for us was in the early morning hours after a big snowstorm. Paul knew I couldn't shovel the snow, then drive to the restaurant, and sit down and eat; therefore, he got up early. He shoveled the driveway while I was in the shower.

We had twice as much snow as anyone else because of the mounds we created for summer planting. When the town plow came down the highway, we felt he accumulated all the snow from the entire street and dumped it at our driveway entrance. I remember several mornings when Paul just finished shoveling, the plow returned just to plug it all up again. Needless to say, we were glad when summer rolled around again.

Winters were hard on us. In cold weather, my body heat escaped faster. The warm, summer air was similar to insulation, and it held the body heat in.

My habits in the winter didn't help the situation.

Paul often said, "You are a worry out there on the highway."

In my comings and goings, I was often alone on the road. Sometimes, when my body temperature dropped, I was the last one to recognize it. And by the time I did, my core temperature might be so low it wouldn't come back up. Paul had seen my body temperature drop severely. He knew the signs. But if Paul was at home, and I was miles away, he couldn't be of any help.

One morning, I was up at daybreak. I did enough shoveling, so my car was able to pull out of the driveway. Then I showered and drove to the restaurant. My skin hurt from being so hot, and my face and ears were extremely red and uncomfortable. I forced myself to eat some breakfast, and three hours later, I was still overheated. But my satisfaction came from trying something new, and I felt it was worthwhile. I stepped out of my regimented behavior into a higher level of confidence. I felt guilty for my husband because he ended up doing all the shoveling, yet he never complained. Occasionally, if we were lucky, Paul hailed a passing snowplow, and they helped us out.

The changing of the seasons, especially the beginning of fall or spring, was rough on my body. It meant the indoor temperatures were also inconsistent and not dependable. The restaurant I went to daily became overly warm. Once I was situated and comfortable with a restaurant, I didn't like changing to another one. I agonized over it for days until my appetite decreased severely, and the migraines increased; then I knew I didn't have a choice. I returned to the other fast food restaurant.

I thought accepting warm conditions was going to be a better way to live. It wasn't long before I realized *too* warm made eating significantly difficult. To help alleviate some of this heat, I brought along a bottle of ice water. I only needed a little bit on my neck, face, and wrists. I wasn't happy sharing this little habit with others; therefore, I nonchalantly walked to the restroom to complete the task. Before long, I was making *three trips* to the restroom to splash cool water on myself prior to eating.

Again, I added another obsession without realizing it. Finally, after months of doing this, I knew I had to stop. I made up my mind to sit still, be calm, think of something pleasant, and *wait* for coolness to happen. This scenario worked, and the bottled ice water ended.

My life in the early nineties: I was home, I was out of the house, I was home, back out, and then home again. In between all of this bouncing around, I cleaned and cooked. And occasionally, I dabbled in some artwork. In the summer, I worked in the garden. The sketching and painting slowed down considerably. I continued to keep the artistic imagination alive with our annual Christmas card.

There was a consistent routine for every meal throughout the year. When Thanksgiving and Christmas appeared on the calendar, the routine changed. On certain holidays, most fast food restaurants were closed. This always presented a problem. And for this reason only, I basically dreaded the holidays. In the past, Paul and I went to a Thanksgiving buffet at one of the hotels. There was plenty of lovely food, and the temperature in the dining room was comfortable.

Over time, they also changed their heating system to forced air. We didn't know about the switchover. Like always, we made our reservations and expected the same conditions. We checked our coats and walked into the dining room; Paul took one look at me. I had a shawl pulled up around my neck. My shoulders were hunched forward trying to get warm, and my hands were clinched together to keep the circulation going. My face turned pale and sad. He knew what the next move was going to be. We walked out the door rather discouraged. Many other nice restaurants also converted to the forced air heating system. I remember one year, we went to so many restaurants we were psychologically a wreck by the time we found one close to suitable. Each year, our list shrunk until we gave up trying.

The holidays became irritating instead of happy. Paul said he would rather stay at home; I could go anywhere that was appropriate. I always prepared Paul's holiday dinner before I left the house. Paul said he didn't care what the process was; as long as I ate a meal, he didn't mind staying at home, waiting for my return.

Where I ended up eating my meal didn't matter, as long as I was out of the house, in warm surroundings, with no moving air. One year, after Paul ate his dinner, he went with me to the Albany Medical Center cafeteria. The walk from where we parked the car to the cafeteria was rather a long distance. By the time I reached my destination, I was extremely warm from all the temperature changes. I was the one who suggested we eat our holiday dinner in the cafeteria, so I didn't have the right to complain. The tension between us increased until I thought I might explode from stress. I was anxious to return home and end the holiday.

Another year, we tried McDonald's on the New York State Thruway. I dreaded the ordeal even before we left the house. I knew, somehow, I would eventually eat somewhere, but there was added stress when another person tagged along, even when it was my husband. I worried about him losing patience with me. From this point forward, I went alone. That way, only one person was miserable. The Albany Airport cafeteria wasn't too bad, and then there was the Holiday Inn Courtyard near the indoor pool. The surroundings were nice, and it was peaceful; no one else was around to make me feel nervous or guilty because I was eating my holiday dinner in an inappropriate setting.

For many years thereafter, I dined at a Stewart's convenience store. The seating area was all right as long as one table was available out of only two tables! I always brought along my trusty canvas bag filled with food from home. At all times, I purchased soda and a hot tea. It was better when the holiday ended. Then I could go back to *my normal* obsessive behavior.

My illness had put a strain on my relationship with my family. I rarely saw my sister, and when I did the moments weren't the same as our childhood days.

In the late 80's we went or separate ways. My addiction altered my ability to make rational choices. I longed for friendship, people to love me, and pieces of my past. However, my behavior put a monumental wedge between us.

There was a void in my life as big as a mountain. I believe the separation was meant to be. God knew when the time would be right for us to empathize with one another. The healthier I became, the more I missed her.

During my daily prayer, I asked God, "Please reunite my sister and me. My heart aches. I miss her terribly."

On Christmas day, in 1991, I prayed one more time. I was nervous, but I picked up the telephone and called her. While the telephone rang, and I was waiting, I felt and heard my heart pounding. I thought it would burst. She answered the phone with a pleasant hello.

I told her who was calling and said, "Please forgive me. I am so sorry. I love you."

She said, "I love you, too."

Then we both burst into tears. The emotion was difficult to bear, and beautiful at the same time. After the moisture dissipated, we continued to talk about our lives.

I thought I had lost her forever. Being reunited with a loved one is truly a special gift.

In the spring of 1992, we made plans for a sister get-together.

After a few visits we asked if my nephew could spend the night. It would be his first night away from her. She agreed. This wasn't a normal event for us because in the past, my addiction to cold water would have interfered. I was too nervous and embarrassed by my compulsive behavior. I didn't want anyone to see me in action. Paul was the only person that really knew my everyday existence. Even my doctor didn't know the extent of my obsession.

My sister didn't give me garments, as gifts, I couldn't wear. For several holidays, she gave me scarves, which added life and a new, spicy, fun look to my appearance. For one Christmas she gave me a sweater vest. Little by little, a change, she wasn't aware of, was happening. I was thrilled with a fashion accessory so different from what I usually wore. I never received too many compliments on my *uniform polyester look*. The scarves, and the vest, from my sister created a stir wherever I went. Her well-thought-out gifts were the beginning of my desire to move away from polyester materials. I didn't think I'd ever see the day when I would wear anything different. She opened my eyes, and my mind, to change — clothing and house décor.

Chapter 26
Stop, Stop, Stop

The strict and persistent routine of eating all my meals in a restaurant continued for a long time — about eleven years or more. Early one morning, in 1993, I finally realized I was totally wiped out. I was tired of packing up the food and driving to a restaurant. I constantly worried about the room temperature and struggled with the blowing air. Never sure of what my body temperature was, I had to check it all the time — and do whatever I had to do in order to keep it up, especially under unfavorable conditions.

My addiction to cold water was gone. Finally, I was in the *warm zone* of life. I had prayed for all of this, and God answered me. Now, I wasn't able to tolerate any moving air at all; a whisper gave me a migraine. At one time, we searched the universe for cold, which was hard to obtain. Now, all establishments we visited had installed new, more efficient heating and cooling systems with excessive moving air. I'm not really sure why the drastic change happened. Possibly, I had put myself into too much cold. Maybe my body was retaliating and preserving itself.

I couldn't tolerate the *every day out of the house* obsessive routine anymore. I was beyond worn-out, and the migraines became intense. The prescription drugs didn't alleviate the pain. The migraines put me to bed, without nourishment, at least, once a month. Each time this happened, it set me back on my weight and my energy level. Over the years, my body stopped *the train* before it crashed. I was never the one to cease the addiction or obsession on my own; some traumatic event always occurred first.

The whole rat race finally ended. I opened my eyes to a new day. After that, my body didn't have the energy to shower, dress, or pack up breakfast and walk out the door.

I said to Paul, "If you agree to fix my breakfast each morning, I will eat all my meals at home. I'm just too tired. I can't live on this schedule anymore."

I was relieved; I didn't have to go anywhere. It was as if a big elephant had been removed from my back. A huge burden was finally gone.

Paul was so surprised I wasn't going to McDonald's. He said, "I'll fix anything you want anytime of the day."

This moment was beautiful. We were on our way to a much better life for both of us.

My entire repetitive behavior had been totally turned upside down. I never wanted to slip back into my old habits or the obsession of eating all my meals in restaurants; this was going to work. Wouldn't it be fantastic to sit down and eat without cooling myself first? I wasn't sure if the transition would be so simple; it would take time. After all, Rome wasn't built in a day. To compensate for being a little apprehensive, I came up with stipulations. If Paul agreed, then I knew some of my fears would be eliminated.

I would have to eat breakfast as soon as I came down to the kitchen.

Paul needed to prepare and serve it.

I could get my own lunch, dinner, and snack, although I required to eat alone.

Paul was thrilled I wanted to stay home and, of course, went along with me. I wanted to be okay in my own home and feel comfortable about eating all my meals there. One way or another, we were going to make this drastic change happen.

I liked conversation. I enjoyed being around people. When it came time to eat, I wanted to be alone, except for breakfast. I was about to eat all my meals at home. I had to forget why I left home in the first place. The concentration had to be on the present, not on the past. I was entering a new era.

It wasn't easy accepting a new routine. First thing in the morning was the most difficult. I was very warm after getting out of bed. Whether I wanted to change or not, the reality was there. The good thing was I was not giving up. There was always a way to work with what I had in front of me. Finally, I came to a conclusion: eating at home was going to become a way of life with no turning back. No one was telling me I had to do this. That was one of the beautiful characteristics Paul possessed. Most of the time, he let *me* decide on the next improvement. By doing it this way, I was able to see how much better my life was going to be. We still had some quirks to get over. When I realized I didn't need them, then more changes would occur.

For a long time, our daily jaunt to a restaurant was close to perfect. I felt as if I were in control of the routine. Each day was as I planned it. That is until the restaurant environment changed. Then our predictable day no longer existed. At the time, I was rather upset. I dwelled on the topic daily. Little did I realize God had a plan for me. Something had to be done so I would move forward and alter my lifestyle. I believe He knew I could do it.

I allowed Paul to eat breakfast with me because he prepared it, and then I was able to sit still and become relatively cool. We continued this for quite some time.

I had a difficult time figuring out why I was so warm when I ate in a house. When people were around me, it was worse; however, I allowed Paul to join me in a restaurant and during one meal at home. I also looked for a lot of space between the walls and me. In my mind, the space transmitted coolness.

Small spaces made me feel closed in. Think how warm it would be inside a small box versus a huge box. When I took a casual walk, I liked the wide-open places. Even our small living room with a cathedral ceiling was not spacious enough. I felt trapped. Entrapment created heat; walking gave me a sense of freedom, which, in turn, cooled my body.

We continued our walks in the local mall. It seemed endless, as if the mall had no boundaries. I loved taking long strides, and with each brisk step, I could feel the air sweep across my body. I became tired before I was warm.

Paul had great difficulty keeping up with me. He often teased me about my gait, especially in the winter when the outdoor pavement was icy. He frequently said, "It is icy and slippery outside; keep those long legs together."

What I was used to doing was about to be modified. The size of my walking area shrank. My dining area became smaller. Once upon a time, this type of alteration made me very nervous. Now I was okay.

I didn't want to be dependent upon Paul for each meal. I was able to prepare all three meals. The only element standing in the way was the never-ending fear of becoming too hot. Paul always had me on his mind, and he certainly wanted me to succeed and to continue eating at home. He was sure this new change would be beneficial.

Paul said, "I will leave you alone in the house to do your own thing. When you are ready, you can prepare your lunch, and then take your time to eat it in peace. I won't be here to interfere or to talk to you. If you have this assurance each day, then maybe it will help you."

I thought Paul's suggestion sounded like a good plan. He left for McDonald's each morning and enjoyed reading the newspaper and drinking several cups of coffee. He stayed a little longer if he found someone to talk with. I was alone in the house; the morning was mine. I took a sigh of relief because I knew I had all the time I needed to prepare myself for lunch. Any activity would boost my appetite; that was a good thing.

In the past, I hesitated to move excessively. The fear of not being able to get rid of body heat scared me. I needed a guarantee for this plan to work. What better way to do it than to have a trial run, especially with no one else around? When I was alone, I usually found a solution. I planned to lie down, be very patient, and stay there as long as I needed to. If I felt cool, then I knew my plan worked, and it was okay to stay at home. Whenever there was a new challenge, I pictured the entire change, step by step, in my mind. This diminished part of the fear and increased my confidence toward the ultimate goal.

I prepared our evening meal, and then I served Paul. After he finished his dinner, he left the kitchen, and I ate by myself. Whatever I suggested, Paul went along with me. He wanted this *home experience* to be as comfortable as possible.

Each morning, as I put my feet on the floor, I was so relieved I didn't have to leave the house. My new lifestyle was a *beautiful thing*. I knew we were going to make it as long as we were in agreement, and we had each other.

I have moments when I make an effort to bring back those days that are stored in my memory bank. I attempt to detach myself from the scene and look at it as purely an observation. I see myself as a young woman who was eager for life but still very cautious. She has overcome some fears but has many more to work through. She is searching for inner peace. She is looking for a place in this world where she can comfortably *stay put* and not look for all her happiness from other people, other places, or other things. She feels the happiness must come from being content within herself and loving God. She will continue to grow and find more freedom than she ever thought possible.

My *new life* opened a door of many possibilities. I enjoyed the liberty of staying home all day if that was what I wanted to. The thought of becoming involved with a project created a spark of enthusiasm. A project would involve creativity and staying focused on something other than my habits. Along with the positive aspects, there were some negative ones.

Working on a project could create more heat in my body than making beds or other household chores. There again, this was an issue that plagued me in the past; however, it was not going to be a problem now. I was ready for the challenge. Running away from heat wasn't going to be my destiny.

In the late afternoon, I generally developed a headache. I no longer had the urge to flee. The headaches were a part of my existence. Sadly, migraines were going to be included in my journey. I had to learn how to cope with them the best I could. Prescription drugs didn't seem to be the answer. I incorporated alternative healing methods into my daily life. They helped ease the pain at times.

When a headache occurred, I compared my body to a snow globe being shaken all day long. The snow had to settle for the scene to become calm. So, in retrospect, I took myself away from everyone and everything in order to *stop*. I knew if I was alone, I could bring my warm body back to a comfortable temperature, thus, enabling me to eat my meals. I only needed about ten to fifteen minutes to lie on my bed before each meal. By removing all thoughts from my mind, I was left in a more peaceful state. The tension and tightness disappeared from my head. This is something that worked well and was harmless. It did take a little time, and Paul needed to wait for me.

Paul always said, "Take your time and relax, so you can enjoy your meal."

I looked forward to these quiet moments. Closing my eyes was very soothing. I talked to God and thanked him for allowing my body to cool without cold water. Eliminating any body movement and clearing the clutter from my mind allowed me to cool down naturally. Eventually, I was able to do this even when it was ninety degrees outside. I could not rush these moments. If I did, then the heat lingered.

Once I was back on my feet, my body was calm, relaxed, and cooler. Then I was able to eat a sufficient amount of food. A few times, I attempted to eat without lying down first; my consumption of food was cut in half.

For me, eating my dinner alone was a way to preserve the calmness I obtained while lying on the bed. And the quiet atmosphere of our home was a change from the chaos of a restaurant. It took many years to get to this point in time; however, here I was. I was amazed I was able to sit and eat a meal without pain and fear. I was content with the direction of my life. God had given me a miracle.

The last time I felt even close to this moment was probably in the early seventies, some twenty years ago. I couldn't count the first couple of years I lived with Paul. Then I ate because I was afraid my body temperature would drop, or Paul might ask me to leave. And most important, I would flat-out die if I didn't put something in my stomach. Now, I was getting closer to a normal way of eating. I didn't have a windstorm over my head or freezing temperatures to increase my appetite. I ate in *a God-given setting of tranquility* without anything to boost my appetite, and it tasted oh so good.

Whether I was eating alone or with Paul, I didn't want to be interrupted during a meal. Paul and I accepted this as a normal requirement in our household. Interruptions only heated me up and interfered with the amount of food I ate. Paul simply told people not to call at mealtime. My stepchildren were empathic and respected this. They asked what time we ate dinner and avoided calling us at that hour. They didn't ask why, and we didn't explain. Most likely, no one would understand, so why bother to explain? It was important to Paul that I ate a sufficient amount, so we were very strict about our request. Paul was on my side and tried to understand, knowing it allowed me to relax and remain cool.

Paul said, "I don't care if the President of the United States comes to visit. Do whatcha gotta do when you gotta do it, and never mind anyone else. Don't let anyone interfere with your eating, not even me."

As far as what I ate, I made sure to continue with a balance of heat-inducing foods with the chilling foods. I ate foods with some fat to make my body feel warm — warm enough to keep the body temperature up. As soon as I felt a little too warm, I ate nonfat foods like carrots, lettuce, cantaloupe, and broccoli, plus I drank a lot of water. This way, my body didn't overheat, and my weight stayed the same.

Eating a dessert, especially ice cream or candy, was out of the question. The ingredients usually contributed to a headache. But fear was also a factor. I related it to the past when one bite was never enough. Sitting down to a simple bowl of ice cream ended in devouring the entire half-gallon. And if that wasn't enough, I continued with more sweets and fats until nothing else fit in my stomach. Binging left a bad taste in my mouth; I didn't want to go there again.

We never had any guests for dinner. If we received any invitations, we declined. It seemed useless to give an explanation, plus it was embarrassing to admit my unusual behavior. This was our problem to work through. Eventually, the invites ceased. What we had was safe, and the progress was good. We didn't want to upset the apple cart right now. The time wasn't right, and when it was, we would know it.

The more time at home, the more projects I became involved in. I wasn't running all over the Capital District. I had a lot of free time in my home, and the only hindrance was the pressing schedule I created within our domain. This opened many possibilities where I was able to develop many abilities. I enjoyed making changes in our decor and putting my own flare throughout each room. Finding new resting places for a multitude of items seems to be my passion. Paul said he didn't mind, even though he constantly loses things because I rearrange the house so often.

I was comfortable with our new, everyday life. It worked out well, so I continued it for years. I had put myself into a safety bubble. If someone talked or, even worse, talked negatively about a topic I didn't want to hear, I wasn't able to eat. I made an agreement with myself; mealtime was going to be a happy time of the day. It would be peaceful and not upsetting. If I had these elements all around me, I would eat all my meals at home forever.

I put terrible restrictions on myself and cut people out of my life by doing this. At the time, my requests seemed very important. I knew I had come a long way, but I still had a ways to go.

At one time, I was eating in my car after submersing myself in frigid water. Now, at least, I was eating in my own home with no cold water. That alone was remarkable.

Paul went along with just about everything; he was thrilled I was eating my meals in our home, even though three of those meals I ate alone.

Finally, my day wasn't taken up with driving all over the place, looking for the perfect restaurant. It had become a nightmare outside our door. There were no perfect places anymore; I could not control their temperatures. I tried, and it was impossible. It was like fighting city hall. At home, I had a better chance of keeping the house at an even temperature, plus I didn't even have to leave the house. Each day, I could decide whether to stay in or go out. The compulsion of "I must get out here" was gone.

Paul agreed to do all the grocery shopping. The dairy department was extremely cold all year. I didn't have to stand still too long before my body temperature dropped, and later, I developed a migraine. He did all the errands — in all directions and in all categories. The less temperature changes I had to endure, the better. I took care of the inside of the house. Our way of life worked for us — and our cats.

I spent most of my days in a warm environment. The pendulum swung from one extreme to another. Paul never figured out how that happened. At one time, I craved cold. Now, I couldn't bear it. During my lifetime, I have endured unpleasant conditions even if I became ill. It was a part of my life.

I made an attempt to avoid the cold and the wind. That was possible because of Paul. He didn't want me to suffer. Occasionally, I ventured out into it, and the end result was usually the same: a migraine and low body temperature.

I am able to bring my body temperature up rather quickly; however, the migraines last a few days or until I adjust myself to the indoor elements.

Maybe over time, I readjusted my thermostat.

Chapter 27
The Girl in the White Hat

October 1978, I arrived at Paul's house not wearing a hat. He almost insisted I wear one. I argued, saying they made me too warm, and I would become ill if I wore a hat. Winter approached, and he just flat-out bought me a hat whether I wanted one or not. It was a chic, beret style. I wore the hat outside *only* and was eager to take it off once indoors. In the summer, I never wore a hat.

In the eighties, I was a regular customer at McDonald's. I chose to sit where there was cool, moving air. It took me an hour to eat my dinner. If I didn't wear a hat, the air made my neck stiff, and I suffered with a headache.

The hat was never a fashion statement. It was solely for protection against the elements and for minimization of the migraines. The hat worked like extra insulation. On most days, the covering helped to keep my body temperature elevated. As I accustomed myself to a hat, removing it left my head cold. The more days I left it on, the more difficult it was to take it off. I could not tolerate any coolness on my head; therefore, I wore a lightweight open-weave hat on cool, summer days — cool being any temperature below eighty degrees. In time, I wasn't able to stop *wearing a hat*. I needed to wear it at all times. I could be butt naked and still needed a hat on my head!

The stares I received were many. People asked why I always had a hat on my head. I have tried eliminating it but to no avail. I soon realized I couldn't let other people's comments interfere with my healing.

I have to focus on what is important. An opinion or catty remark isn't worth getting upset over. Without the hat, the migraines become worse. I often pray for a life without a hat. I know the hat will come off when it's supposed to.

My first hat was an angora beret. It tended to be a bit warm indoors; therefore, I bought another hat. This one was the infamous *white hat*. It was a medium-weight knit, suitable for in and out of the house. Luckily, I bought three of them. It wasn't long before I needed to wear two hats at the same time on wintry days: the angora beret and the white knit. The indoor hat was the most difficult to find. Certain materials were too warm to wear indoors.

Paul and I were always on the lookout for a copy of the white hat. When we walked through a store, we almost always ended up in the hat department. After trying on several hats, I was sure I found the right one. The amount of time I wore it in the store was too brief. The real assessment had to be made at home. Never knowing the *supply or demand* and if the hat would still be in the store at a later date, I put stress on myself to purchase something. On top of that, I bought more than one, just in case I couldn't find a hat elsewhere. Even after finding a hat, I was never sure how long it would last on my head.

The only true test was to wear it every minute of the day for several days. If I didn't feel too hot or too cold, then the hat passed the trial. Out of all the hats I ever bought, the infamous white hat *was and is* my favorite. Seasons change, and so do hat styles. After I found the white hat, every year thereafter, not one store had the same exact hat. The style existed but not the fabric. I knew my white hat wouldn't last forever. I continued to buy the style even though the material was a little bit different. I now have a closet full of unused hats.

I am still wearing those three original white hats almost twenty years later. It seems almost impossible a hat could last that long. I made them last. They stretched, so I added a safety pin in the back. They became thinner and thinner and close to falling apart. I continue to wear them. I was so insistent over a hat; I created an obsession to the white hat.

Without this specific hat, I have difficulty eating and functioning. Any other hat I buy is too warm or not warm enough. I develop a headache, and I just end up removing it and going back to the *white hat*. I look at it in dismay. I know I have to buy a new one. I put hats on my shopping list, have purchased several, and end up right back with the old, white hat.

Intermittently, it is very depressing. I know they do nothing for my appearance, and I truly want to be rid of them. Summer is a tremendous relief. My head feels free to breathe, and it isn't being *held captive with an elastic band*. On warm, summer days, when it is over eighty degrees outdoors, I remove *all* hats. It is magnificent — an *a-ha moment*, for sure.

In the winter, the white hat never comes off. It is worn continuously all day, all night, and even during sex. In the shower, it comes off and is replaced with a shower cap. My head is covered at all times. If the hat slips off during the night, I awake with a migraine. Whenever I need to remove my white hat for a medical test, there is always cause for much concern and stress. Sometimes, on windy days, a third hat is worn, or a scarf is added.

Over the years, as I continued to evaluate my body's reaction to different temperatures, I believe the long-term use of extreme cold water and cold air has played a part in the reason why I become ill in cold surroundings. When I first started swimming, my head was exposed all the time, winter and summer. I even wrapped my head in a cold, wet towel after taking a cold shower. Then I proceeded to walk into the cold outdoors and sit in a cold car to eat my meal. So in those times, my head was certainly exposed to more cold than is normal. This wasn't a one-time event; I exposed my head to cold temperatures day after day after day all winter long.

Chapter 28
More Progress

In 1989, we continued with more renovations. My stepson was very good at taking on just about any construction job. Paul measured up for the materials needed. Most of the time, Paul and I had an idea of what we wanted as the final look. Paul and his son made it all happen. They installed cedar shake siding and a cedar shake roof. One day, I asked if I could place a few boards under the kitchen window. They showed me how it was done, and I went at it with hammer in hand. I was surprised to see the installed board lookin' pretty darn good. We kidded around, saying I could become quite the handyman. The best part was it showed me I was able and willing to take on most any task.

My stepson also renovated our bathrooms. I was sent to the home improvement stores to compare prices and purchase the lighting fixtures and accessories. This was a new avenue on my *life map*. I became totally involved in the renovations, and it created a thirst for doing more of the same.

The little bit I was involved in started a long trend of believing in my ability to master most anything. I was ready for more difficult projects. Each job added to my self-assurance. Paul had given me time to heal, time to grow, and time to find my way. What developed from all of this were freedom, choice, and a meaningful existence. Back in the seventies, when I spent my entire day swimming, I never dreamed a life like this was possible.

We scheduled all construction for late morning. Paul told his son I needed to be alone while eating lunch. To give me more time, they went to McDonald's for breakfast. I ate an early lunch before they returned. I'm not sure any other contractor would have gone along with this, but my stepson was very accommodating. Occasionally, my timing was off, and they were ready to start work before I ate. Again, they went along with me as much as possible by being busy elsewhere on the property. Then I rushed lunch before anyone passed through the kitchen. There were times when it was pertinent for them to pass by me; it couldn't be avoided unless the job was put on hold. Over time, I found myself accepting the challenge as long as no one sat down and talked. I preferred to be alone, but if it didn't work out that way, I was beginning to allow it. I continued with my lunch and realized I was okay. Each time, the interruption was a little easier; however, I wasn't ready for company on a daily basis.

Over time, I gave *the workmen* the green light. They were allowed to begin work whenever they wanted to. Making that adjustment wasn't easy for me. Paul's son was wonderful; he didn't make a big deal out of my obsessive behavior.

For years, we avoided renovating the bathroom because it might be out of commission for a day. Going from one floor to another created a temperature change; therefore, I avoided using the bathroom on the lower level of the house as much as possible, especially during the night or early morning. Paul honored this and understood.

Finally in 1993, we decided to start the demolition. Paul assured me I'd have the bathroom back for morning and evening use. He and his son worked all day with hardly a break, and before evening, the toilet was temporarily back in service. The next day, the toilet was removed from the bathroom, and the bathtub was installed. And once again, the toilet was reinstalled in the evening. Further construction was done in the bathroom the following day, and the toilet was uninstalled again. This continued until the bathroom was far enough along to leave the toilet installed.

Whatever I needed, Paul was always in agreement, and his son never questioned why. I didn't talk with my stepson about my addiction or illness. I'm sure he knew something happened in my past. None of that appeared to matter. He accepted me for who I was at the moment. And because of his understanding, I was okay in carrying out my routine when he was around. For years, Paul was the only one who saw my daily obsessions. The outside world had a sneak peek but nothing like it really was.

Whenever I asked my stepson to do anything around the house, he was there for us. He did all the renovation work for years, moved furniture, worked on plumbing and electric, weeded the garden, picked up heavy objects — for example, granite urns and concrete statues — and moved them to a new location in the garden. I think he came close to renovating every inch of our house. He gave up many of his weekends and saved us a lot of money. But most of all, he allowed me to grow. I looked forward to his arrival every time work was scheduled. The day was brighter when he was there, and I know Paul enjoyed spending time with his son.

Something else added a great deal of pleasure to my life over the years. After a car hit Keefer, we no longer wanted the cats to run free, and yet we continued to adopt more furry kids. All of our *children* were eager to go outdoors. I liked the idea of letting them out into the fresh air; but first, and foremost, we wanted them to be safe. Paul bought cat harnesses. I reinforced them with extra straps so they couldn't wiggle out of them. Our family was growing.

My love of cats was intense. Whenever they crossed my path, and especially if they were in trouble, they stole my heart.

Paul and I both gravitated to the needy. Stray cats drifted into our garden on a regular basis. They probably knew when they found a good thing. We didn't let any of the hungry cats pass by without a meal. Some moved on, and others returned daily.

The cats became my children; the bond between all of us was immeasurable. I could tell them my troubles, my fears, my joys, and my secrets. They loved me unconditionally. My cats taught me many things, and they contributed to my healing. Cats are certainly unpredictable, and so is life.

I found their sense of timing wasn't always the same as mine. At times, they needed tending to right on the spot, not when I finished my obsessive behavior. This was definitely a beneficial life lesson.

I had an addiction to cold water. When I kicked that, other obsessions still existed. For as long as I needed them, Paul never made me stop doing what I thought I had to do. He knew in time they would leave.

I compared the new me to that of peeling an artichoke. I had produced layers of obsessions. Now I was removing one at a time. If I stayed strong in my faith, I would reach the desired center fruit — the fruit of a complete, delightful life.

I truly believed the addiction to cold water was behind me; nevertheless, I stayed away from all swimming areas. Did this indicate I was actually safe? Time would tell.

My mother taught me how to sew when I was quite young. This was another avenue I wanted to dip into and explore my creativity. Paul purchased an inexpensive sewing machine; window curtains and throw pillows started the ball rolling. I bought an older style mannequin from a store going out of business. I didn't use any patterns. Instead, I sketched out the look I wanted, took some measurements, and jumped into action. I continued to study my mannequin and just knew I could design a few outfits. The first one was a Mrs. Santa Claus dress trimmed with fake fur. The mannequin and I were about the same size. On Christmas Day, I wore the outfit to my sister's house to surprise her son. Something special happened as I slipped into the dress — as if I were a character in a storybook. Just for a short moment, I enjoyed being transformed into a different element. We also decorated the garden for Halloween, Easter, and Christmas. The people were constructed out of wire. I knew in my head what I wanted each one to wear, and I went from there. Part of the outfit was gathered from household garments; the rest were handmade.

Little by little, my life was becoming whole again. The migraines continued, but they didn't stop me. I was determined to live my life to the fullest. Unfortunately, instead of quitting when I was tired, I continued to work. I wanted to accomplish as much as possible, but sometimes, my surroundings were too cold. I believe I ended up in bed because my body's defense mechanism was protecting me. I never gave in easily or went to bed to avoid a situation.

When I wasn't able to be on my feet any longer, due to the horrible throbbing pain in my head, that was the only time I curtailed my obsessive-compulsive behavior. Lying in bed wasn't pleasant either. It wasn't a restful seventeen hours; the pain saw to that. If I had my druthers, bed was the last place I wanted to be.

There is something magical and peaceful when viewing an assortment of beautiful flowers. I don't think there is ever a time when too much beauty is objectionable. Each summer, I added flowers to the garden. Paul and I both agreed it was gorgeous. I claimed I had enough flowers; however, each spring I managed to squeeze in a few more. There is something magical and peaceful when viewing an assortment of beautiful flowers. I don't think there is ever a time when too much beauty is objectionable. I drove Paul crazy moving the plants around. Each season I convinced him by saying, "This is something all gardeners do; it is part of gardening."

My grandmother was a gardener. Anyone who gazed upon her lovely garden knew she had a *green thumb*. When I was a little girl, gardening didn't interest me at all. I loved to admire the flowers and smell their beautiful fragrance. Perspiring under the hot sun without a lake nearby — that wasn't my cup of tea.

How time can change so many things; spending time with Mother Earth is enjoyable. Each spring, as the flowers go into full bloom, we are rewarded by their magnificence, and the backbreaking work is definitely worthwhile.

Paul appreciated the flowers as much as I did — maybe more. When I met him, every time we went for a drive, he made sure I looked at all the beauty growing alongside the road, even if most of greenery was considered weeds. Someone once told me anything you don't like could be called a weed. I guess that is why I never considered the roadside flowers weeds.

When I became *a stay at home gal,* every day for over ten years, you would have found an arrangement of Alstroemerias in our home. Paul knew they were my favorites. Their grace and elegance brought peace and harmony to whatever room I placed them. The flowers last for weeks unless you have cats like mine. They began eating them. My babies' health was more important than the flowers.

Presently, we enjoy an assortment of flowers each spring, summer, and fall when we look at our garden. During the winter months, we admire them as a screensaver on the computer.

One hot, summer day in 1996, I was working in my garden when I felt excessively warm. My face was flushed, and the heat in my body was much more than usual. I felt several sores on my lip, and I tried to ignore the signs of an illness. I had so much work to do in the garden, and this wasn't a good time to be sick. I made believe the sores didn't exist. I feverishly stayed with the work to be done, hoping the sores would disappear. I'm not one to give in to ill health easily, but when the nausea started and my head was throbbing, I didn't have a choice. I had to take my temperature. The digital reading was 103 degrees. For me with a normal body temperature of 97 degrees, this reading was a bit much. I had three sore and ugly lumps on my lip. I had put my symptoms off way too long. It was time to be checked by a doctor. Paul and I went to a *walk in* medical practice. I felt so awful I didn't mind the wait. I needed help. The diagnosis was herpes. My eyes grew wide, and I took a deep breath. This wasn't possible. I knew nothing about it, but it still wasn't possible. I was devastated.

As usual, I had negative thoughts racing around in my head. Paul wouldn't want to have sex with me because of this condition. How did I contract it? Would I always have herpes? Would I give it to him? Would the medicine give me a migraine? How long will I feel sick with this infection? All these ideas rushed into my head. The day had been ruined.

When we were finally back in the car, I sat there and cried. Paul couldn't figure out why I was so upset. To me, it seemed awful. I had heard about herpes, but I didn't think I would ever get it. We immediately purchased the medicine. In a very short time, I started to feel better. I told Paul I didn't want to cook supper. I suggested frozen dinners from the market.

Once we were back home, Paul expected the usual. I would eat alone after I fixed his meal. I set the table in the living room, not in the kitchen. I prepared the table with two place settings. He was in another room watching television and didn't see what was going on. For some reason, I didn't feel like eating alone or being by myself. The prognosis wasn't that bad, but I felt my body had betrayed me. I lay down briefly before dinner. When I felt calm and relatively cool, I came back to the table and called Paul.

Paul walked into the living room and remarked, "What is this nice surprise?"

I said, "We are eating dinner together."

We sat for a moment to savor this special occasion. Then Paul said grace and thanked God for this moment, and we enjoyed a wonderful dinner.

I had placed an unpleasant restriction on our eating arrangement. At this monumental dinner, I turned a negative into a positive. We were moving forward, now eating two meals with each other.

I truly believe many things are meant to be. Maybe I wasn't supposed to contract herpes; however, in this case, it caused a significant turn of events. A day that had gone bad was now terrific. We were dining as one. This medical diagnosis didn't take us farther apart like I anticipated; it brought us closer together. I surprised myself when I sat down at the table and began to eat. It felt good. I wasn't on fire. I was okay. This was a moment I would never forget.

From that day forward, we enjoyed dinner together. It became a special part of the day. Paul said there was nothing more important than mealtime. No matter what he was doing, he stopped to eat. If someone took the time to prepare it, then it was only right to show some appreciation. It was pleasant mixing conversation with a meal. The food seemed to taste better. We had a lot to be thankful for.

I became obsessed with being busy. The balance wasn't there. When I had a project to look forward to day after day, I felt more fulfilled and, probably, secure, too. When I worked in the garden, did some sewing, or painted a room, I went full speed ahead. I found it difficult to stop or lighten up. I continuously pushed my limit to get the project down. I also looked for perfection. By putting that much pressure on myself, I gave myself a migraine. Paul often said that once the job was finished, I'd have nothing to do, so why not take it easy. He would normally see what was occurring before I did. Over and over, he cautioned me, saying I worked too hard, and I found it necessary to latch onto something where I'm constantly busy.

Then I'd reply, "That's who I am. Busy makes me happy."

I believe, deep down, I wanted to be content to sit and do nothing for long periods of time. But I wasn't sure if it would ever happen.

My stepson had one of the earliest personal Macintosh computers by Apple Incorporated. Paul was at his house, helping him with a plumbing problem. His son sent the computer home with Paul. And knowing me, he was sure I'd take an interest in it someday. Most of the time, when I thought about sitting in one place for an extended amount of time, I put up a mental block and gave many negative reasons why I wouldn't last. This was different. There was something very intriguing about this little machine. I thought I'd give it a try. I was mesmerized and fascinated, and that allowed me to sit much longer than usual.

I took a typing course in high school, and now it was a blessing. I also read and learned and asked and read some more. Before long, I was creating web pages. The computer was a fantastic diversion. It created a spark of enthusiasm in an area of my brain that had been unused for some time.

There was joy, and there was certainly aggravation in this new experience. It brought the world closer to me, and it expanded my creativity to a level I never dreamed of.

The migraines continued for various reasons, but I didn't give up the computer. I was hooked. I definitely acquired a new habit; however, I thought the computer was a *good* obsession. And there was a huge amount of infinite possibilities ahead.

The computer brought my photography to a new height. It meant sharing photos with friends and relatives. I was inspired to take more silly and fun shots, because I could see the results quickly. Christmas 1997, Paul and I dressed in old, fur coats. The photo was so good we used it for our Christmas card. One person thought it meant we didn't have any heat in the house! The idea was to have fun and to be different. The cats were great subjects for photos, too. Everything in our life seemed to merit a photo. It became a great hobby, and the photo albums continue to document our memories.

When I was constantly swimming or bathing in cold water, that area of the photo album is empty. Paul and I are making up for the lost time by capturing as many moments as possible. On the other hand, it took the bad years to get to the good years. Everything has a place in time, and without it, I believe God would not have brought me to Paul.

Chapter 29
New Century, New Me

The year was 2000.

In the twenty-two years Paul and I were together, no one was invited to our home for a meal. On November 23, 2000, I set five places at the table for Thanksgiving dinner. It had always been a holiday we shared with just the two of us. I asked Paul if we could invite some friends. He thought it would be too much work for me. I insisted and told him I could handle the day just fine.

We had a traditional Thanksgiving dinner. I used my oven for the first and only time. Years ago, when I turned on the oven, the kitchen was engulfed in heat. It gave me a migraine, and I couldn't eat. I bought a convection oven and refrained from using my main oven ever again until this day. I was blessed that the weather was a cold five degrees. And with a window opened a crack, we controlled the temperature of the room. I knew one thing: I wanted to put together a dinner similar to what it was when Mom did all the cooking. I baked breads and pies, made stuffing, and cooked apples for homemade applesauce. Paul was in charge of cleaning the turkey and basting it once it was in the oven.

The table was decorated in Mom's style, pleasing to the eye. The holiday meal was a success. It remains a memorable holiday because it was another breakthrough in changing my routine. The meaning of the holiday was intensified because Paul and I shared the day with friends, and we were thankful for such wonderful blessings bestowed upon us all.

I was at home almost every day, and Paul and I were in an unchangeable routine for the most part. My ingenious projects always gave me a spark of rejuvenation, but I thought we both needed some fun outside the house to perk us up a bit. The drawback, which always entered my thoughts, was the temperature inside a building and the moving air. In order to improve the quality of my life, I needed to thrive inside and outside of the house. Paul had given up so much for me. I felt bad we didn't do more things together outside our home.

Proctor's Theater is located in Schenectady, New York, and they have Broadway shows throughout the year. During the Christmas holiday, the theater presents a special stage production. We had never seen it. Paul worried about my body temperature whenever I left the house in cold weather; therefore, I didn't let him in on what I was planning. This gift was going to be a total surprise. If he had too much time to think about it, I was afraid my good energy would be altered by his negative thoughts. This was going to be our night; I could sense it.

I was finally content in my home, but it was time to reach out and explore new territories. I knew Paul wanted to protect me from any pain and suffering, yet I was ready to take on another challenge. Paul thought the temperatures always created problems for us; therefore, it was easier to stay home. I wanted to spread my wings and make a memory.

I hired a limousine. Two days before the *date night*, I told Paul about the event. He appeared to be somewhat happy. The day arrived, and by nightfall, it was two degrees. We bundled up and walked outdoors. It was a beautiful, clear, starlit evening; and the snow crunched like piles of crackers underfoot. It was breathtaking as we stepped into the limousine. We settled in, and I thought it seemed rather chilly. The driver told us the heat wasn't working in the area around the backseat. I was more than a little upset. Paul was concerned about my body temperature and said maybe we should cancel. Not on your life. I was ready for the night. We were going to the performance. It was too late to call for another car, and somehow we would *wing it*. Paul and I snuggled up to each other. We hoped his body heat would be enough for both of us. We told the driver I had low body temperature. He turned up the heat and the blower in the front section of the limousine. I eagerly waited and prayed this dilemma wouldn't ruin the night. Some warm air filtered to the back, and we managed okay.

The evening was delightful. I saw the entire concert, and the next day, I didn't have a migraine. We survived the night. Another accomplishment added in my journey, and a good one.

That same Christmas holiday Paul and I enjoyed the day with my sister, and her family, in Connecticut. I made it a rule to never leave the house before an early lunch. With two meals under my belt, in the right temperature setting, I had a better chance of eliminating a migraine. Eating lunch outside our home was never an option. I wasn't comfortable eating in restaurants anymore; it was too much of a hassle with the air temperature. We normally stayed at my sister's for an hour or less. Each year, I wanted to visit a little longer; however, I kept my eye on the clock — as if I were Cinderella — only I needed to be back home in Albany around four o'clock. I was told, and believed it, a consistent meal schedule is important for anyone who suffers from migraines. We often cut our visit short in order to stay on my timetable.

This holiday, we didn't realize how late it was, and when we glanced at the time, we were amazed it was well after four. I knew there was a restaurant/inn nearby, and my sister confirmed it was open. We said our good-byes and were a little sad because our wonderful day was ending. As soon as Paul and I were seated in the car, I surprised him.

I asked, "Do you want to eat dinner in Connecticut?"

Paul was quite pleased. He said, "You never cease to amaze me."

I was eager to add another challenge. The inn was elegantly decorated for the holidays with an old-fashioned charm that oozed from every room. The temperature was perfect, and without any moving air, I was content and comfortable. As I sat next to my husband, I felt complete. I wanted the moment to be frozen in time so we could savor it just a little while longer.

Since I was incorporating new adventures into my life, my mind was free to wander and dream. While eating my lunch one summer afternoon, I had a brainstorm. Wouldn't it be wonderful to water ski one more time?

In the summer of 2001, I went water skiing at the age of fifty-four!

Because I grew up on a lake, it was a great opportunity to learn how to water ski. My father was an excellent teacher. The first time I made it up on skis, the feeling took my breath away.

There is something so free about gliding across the water with your feet on two flat pieces of wood, the wind in your hair, and a fine mist hitting your face while you feel as if you are soaring through the air. On a hot, summer day, there was nothing like it.

My memories kept bugging me until I made up my mind to water ski again. The air blowing in my hair didn't excite me now; I would wear a bathing cap. Back then, I used to drop one ski upon leaving the dock. I wasn't sure I'd be up to that at fifty-four. My family's cabin had been sold years ago, but my cousin owned a cabin on Copake Lake.

My ties to the lake were gone; only the memories were left. I learned to ski behind my uncle's boat, and now my cousin owned it. In my daydreaming, I pictured myself behind this grand boat one more time. And I felt young and foolish once again.

My cousin and I were communicating via the computer and sharing many photos of our past. He invited Paul and me to visit him at the lake anytime we wanted to. When I came up with this wondrous idea of water skiing, it just happened to be around Paul's birthday, which is in August, and normally, that month is warm. We decided to celebrate Paul's birthday at the lake. Paul didn't have a clue what I had in mind; again, he would have worried too much. I asked my cousin if he could take me skiing. I was extremely active and in good shape, so why not give it a shot? Isn't it said that life begins at fifty?

I was acquiring this free-spirited attitude; it was time for me to blossom. I think when I told Paul, he thought I was kidding. The day could have been warmer, which was Paul's concern. I wore an extra shirt over my bathing suit, put on the life jacket, and slipped into the skis. I was up on the first try. The thrill was beyond exhilarating; it was a natural high. I was in a state of genuine happiness. All went well until I decided to go over the boat's wave. Coming back, I caught an edge and flipped forward face first into the water.

When my cousin brought me back to the dock, I was as white as a ghost from the cold water. My body temperature was ninety-four degrees. After many hugs and congratulations, I quickly dressed and sat in my car with the heater on full blast. My body temperature needed to be elevated even before I drove the car out of the parking lot. Paul said he was terribly concerned about me out there in the cold water. I wasn't even thinking about it. First of all, I had just put on a pair of water skis at the age of fifty-four. As I was swimming towards the dock, I realized something even more important.

Finally, after thirty years, I knew at that very moment the addiction to water was gone — I could swim or not swim; it didn't matter. I'm not sure how I knew it, but deep down in my soul, I felt different. I wasn't tempted for the "one more swim on another day," just because I went into the water.

I developed a bad migraine from the cold water and the wind blowing on me. It kept me up all night, but I didn't care. The mere thought of me water skiing once again made it all worthwhile. Granted, my posture was terrible. It wasn't even close to my teenage years. The perfect form wasn't as important as hanging on to the ski rope. My life was moving in the right direction.

While in the water, I thought, "Water, you don't have a hold on me anymore. I won the battle. I am triumphant."

If I was to swim for relaxation on a daily basis, I'm not sure what would happen. From what I am told, an addiction is never gone. But for now, I think I am safe. That last dip in the water was good enough for me. At the time, I wanted to hold on to the positive thoughts and then float in the satisfaction of conquering this awful addiction.

Another summer came and went. The transition from one season to another wasn't my favorite time of the year. The temperature changes continued to cause migraines. However, I continued to improve.

A very unexpected invite came our way. We were asked to Christmas dinner. A very dear friend knew that at one time, I only ate in restaurants and now, in my own home, but she wanted to give me the opportunity. My initial instinct was to decline. I didn't want to let go of my old secure patterns; they gave me comfort and security. I was being smothered by my lifestyle, but the familiarity of my ways was tolerable compared to trying something so drastically new. I wanted to say yes, for Paul more than myself.

Before the day arrived, Paul asked me several times what I had planned. I couldn't give him an answer. I wanted to; I just wouldn't commit to it. I was afraid, yet I wanted this wonderful occasion to happen. Before I changed any part of my familiar behavior, I closed my eyes and pictured it step by step. I couldn't see the future; however, that was what I was trying to do. I wanted to make sure I would survive any new experience.

This invitation was part of my recovery toward a new life. Change is possible, and our friend was placed in my path for this reason. She told us we could wait until Christmas Day to decide. I didn't want to pass it up, yet it wasn't something I could make a decision on instantly. We spent the day with my sister, in Connecticut, as usual. Paul frequently told me it was fine if we ate at home just like all the other years; the decision was totally up to me. I didn't know myself what I was going to do. All the way back to Albany, I planned on eating at home. I believe making such an assessment took away any stress. That awful thing called fear builds up in my mind so easily.

We were about three minutes from our home. I said to Paul, "Let's join our friend for dinner. I want to see if I can *pull it off.*"

The house was decorated beautifully. The aroma coming from the kitchen smelled like home cooking, and my taste buds began to come alive. I did lie down on her couch before dinner. I was still afraid to sit at the table without cooling myself first. Everyone seemed to accept my behavior as natural, so I felt right at home.

All the wonderful dishes that our friend prepared tasted marvelous. Needless to say, we enjoyed the holiday meal. Paul and I were rather overwhelmed with how the day ended; I had accepted a new challenge and moved past my fears. We were exceedingly happy. This day was a gift from God and perfect from start to finish.

These special events were major breakthroughs. And I did have time to prepare *myself* prior to the day.

On the other hand, if someone happened to stop in on the *spur of the moment*, normally, I would have dropped a hint that we were ready to eat or wait until they left, before Paul and I ate our dinner. And as the time grew closer to our *normal* eating hour, the stress would have escalated.

On this memorable evening, in 2007, I was busy, and dinner wasn't on time. Dr. Howard arrived unannounced. Years ago, her timing would have upset me and caused a great deal of stress. On this particular evening, I didn't even think anything of it. I'm glad I didn't, because I admire and respect Dr. Howard. And later on, I would have felt horrible if this evening had turned out differently. God gave me an instant vision to put my normal behavior aside and include Dr. Howard. I just grabbed a third plate and set the table for another person. There was ample pork on the grill. I put an extra potato in the oven. There was plenty of salad, and luckily, I had just made a pumpkin cake. I assembled the meal rather quickly, and it was pretty darn good. Dr. Howard's presence made it taste even better. What I experienced on that evening had been missing from my life for too long. After these several instances, I am totally fine with people *popping in* when I am eating a meal. I can't even describe how fantastic that is.

My hair was short for over fourteen years. I held on to the thought that short hair equals coolness. I had refused to let it grow long. With a new century and a new me, I yearned for variations in my life — a new life. This would be a good time for a refreshing hairstyle. It was fun to watch the change and how it made me feel. Pretty, sexy, and more stylish. Hats looked great. My whole appearance changed. The hair on my neck was an asset. It kept away any draft, and my neck stayed warmer. When I went outside on frigid, wintry days, I didn't mind the cold as much.

In the years to come, I took up painting again. Only, this time, the brush was on the wall and not the paper. The new approach was exhilarating, and I was eager to prove to myself I could accomplish a big undertaking. Especially one Paul and I would have to look at for years to come.

One day, after I just finished painting the walls in the lower bedroom, I was too tired to cook. I suggested a pizza delivery. This was something we had never done. I had put myself on a restricted diet with as little fat as possible. The fat in food heated me up too much. I was accustomed to this diet that rarely changed.

Paul said, "Your diet is out of whack today."

The thought of doing something totally different without knowing the outcome was awesome. And to top it off, we shared a beer. I didn't think about the possibility of a binge; I just enjoyed it.

What an eye opener that was. I realized I could tolerate foods higher in fat by ending the meal with the same items I used to counteract any warmth I felt when eating all my other meals, for example: raw vegetables, fresh fruit and always plenty of water. The only difference was that with the foods higher in fat, I had to eat more of the cooling foods. At this point, we could change our menu around and break up the *sameness*.

As it turned out, I ended up painting every room in the house. From that point on, I had a thirst for home improvement projects. As soon as I finished one project, I looked around for another area that needed a facelift.

Paul taught me how to use a drill and a chop saw. The first time I held the drill, I was very nervous and afraid of ruining the wood. Paul was patient and kept telling me I was doing fine. He had always been the one to use the power tools. I was a little intimidated; however, I wanted to learn. Cutting wood trim and baseboards was a little tricky. I managed after some figuring and frustration. We purchased four unfinished solid wood doors. Hiring someone else to refinish any wood product can be quite costly. I was sure I could do the job myself, if I put my mind to it.

Paul and his son installed a wood floor years ago. We never coated it with polyurethane. I thought if I could refinish the doors, I could certainly work on the floor. Paul was a very good teacher with years of experience and knowledge. He was my inspiration when it came to do-it-yourself home repairs or improvements. In twenty-eight out of the thirty-two years that I have known Paul, he always did ninety-eight percent of the work himself.

Over time, I needed less assistance. The challenge, the accomplishment, and the end result were rewarding and satisfying. Plus it saved money. I believe women can do almost anything they put their mind to.

The one project I'm still not thrilled with is installing a toilet. We had a leaky one no matter what we did. That isn't my favorite job. There aren't too many projects or fix-it jobs I won't attempt. I do leave the plumbing and electric to a professional.

More than once, Paul said, "You are my biggest accomplishment in life."

The computer brought positive changes into my life. I am able to sit still, and that is a very good addition to my lifestyle. Instead of using a canvas for painting, I use a computer software program to create my drawings. The computer offers many challenges and keeps me on my toes — a great way to exercise the brain mixed with enjoyment.

The Internet is responsible for some of my most important friendships, too. In 1999, while surfing the Internet, I was searching for someone to e-mail. I came across Ms. Sunshine. I loved the name. I knew I wanted to contact her. We wrote several e-mails back and forth. Before we knew it, days turned into years. We were compatible right from the start. The first time we talked was on the Internet. As soon as I heard her voice and laughter, I smiled. Her positive energy transformed any unpleasant moment into a wonderful day.

Her e-mails were so upbeat and positive; I looked forward to them each day. Ms. Sunshine is an intuitive counselor. She is also extremely gifted in *people energy*, which is what I call it. Besides being my friend, she also took the place of a psychotherapist in my life. She never tried to force me to change my ways. Her knowledgeable approach and her way with words conveyed the message. When I was alone and quiet, her voice lingered in my head. I recognized that her abilities were powerful. She knew how to help people with their issues; it just took me time to realize it.

We had several therapy *sessions* on the telephone. I complained and talked about what was bothering me. She listened and gave her thoughts on each situation. She didn't just tell me what I wanted to hear. In fact, sometimes, she made me realize things I never noticed about myself. I wasn't always sure about her solutions. And darn it, she was continuously right. I say that in a constructive manner.

Ms. Sunshine amazed me with her intuitiveness. One of our discussions was about my need to control. I never realized it was so bad until she pointed out some instances. She helped me whittle the controlling personality down to some degree. Then I was less stressed and had fewer headaches. She seemed to know what I was thinking or how I was feeling most of the time. Her counseling helped me to recognize my inappropriate approach to irritating circumstances.

She told me to take a step backward, count to ten, and wait before reacting to an unpleasant situation. If I was controlling someone or something, then it was time to back off. When I told her I had to stay on a rigid schedule, again, she told me it was a form of controlling or being in charge. As long as I allowed this, I would never grow.

One evening, she and I talked a long time. I love talking with her, and on this particular evening, I felt really good. I went with the flow, never looking at the time. It was after midnight when we finished talking. I try not to do this because then I am wide-awake and can't go to sleep. Since I didn't go to bed until late, I was exhausted the next morning.

Normally, when I'm tired, I continue through the day, not giving in to take a nap, especially in the morning. I couldn't risk sleeping through lunch. Around nine-thirty in the morning, I had to lie down. The next thing I knew, it was noon. When I awoke, I was shocked that I had fallen asleep. Usually, I eat lunch at ten, never wavering. I was way off my schedule, and if lunch were late, then dinner would be, too. There had to be so many hours between lunch and dinner.

Typically, if my pattern was disrupted, I would have been painfully upset and mad for allowing myself to falter. Instead, I dressed and ate my lunch. The rest of the day went well. I believe it was from adequate rest and being relaxed.

When I relayed this event to my friend, she replied, "See, you can mix things up a little. Don't try to control the day; go where it takes you. I think you will be happier if you do that with many situations. Let go and let God."

I had survived unintentionally changing the day around. It turned out remarkably better than most. She has helped me to grow and try new things in my life. Ms. Sunshine is very supportive and holds a special place in my heart. She has played a big role in my *coming back into the real world*. All I need is to hear her voice on the telephone, and my day is brighter. The energy she projects is very therapeutic and healing.

In 2006, my Internet friend boarded a plane from out west and flew to Albany. She stayed with Paul and me for five days. We talked about this for months before it happened. I was excited until I accepted the reality. Then I was fearful. Most visitors are only with us for an hour or two. Ms. Sunshine was coming to stay for five days.

I wanted assurance that my strict routine would continue even with someone new in the house. I was easing up on the specific eating schedule, yet I didn't drift too far away from it. I felt confident she would understand all my *oddities*. After deciding yes and then no and back to yes, which continued for many months, I finally gave in. I was somewhat anxious, yet I wanted to meet my friend in person and spend time with her. She was a wonderful houseguest and went along with everything. When I wanted time to eat my lunch alone, she and Paul left the house and went to Wal-Mart or found an ice cream shop. If I wasn't able to sit still and talk, she read while I did my *thing*. I couldn't have asked for anyone better to share in this new undertaking. The day she departed, I cried my eyes out.

Since Ms. Sunshine's visit, I am more adaptable to situations. Thank God, I am more flexible in my everyday life than I was in the past. It is terrible to be a slave to anything unless it is a medical problem where a specific schedule is needed to maintain staying alive.

After attempting many indoor projects, I moved outdoors. In 2007, my stepson installed concrete pavers in the front of our home. The concrete sidewalk was disintegrating. It was in need of much repair. Instead of installing another of the same, we thought concrete pavers would cost less money and add more character to our entrance. Once I saw how beautiful it looked, my mind went on overdrive. I suggested we expand the pavers. Before we knew it, half of the front yard was being taken over with the new look. The work was exhausting but beautiful. I could see the project was a lot for one person. After watching my stepson, I proceeded to install concrete pavers on a small area.

The following summer, I installed a back patio and a low stonewall and covered two stoops all with concrete pavers. I used a caulking gun to glue the caps, caulk windows and doorways, and fill in concrete cracks. No one could stop me now! Every project was attacked with vigorous determination and, sometimes, overtaxed my body, which can be a flaw. Thank God, my body eventually stops me and shouts, "Hey, I need a break." The stonework resulted in two total hip replacements. Both hipbones were in bad shape before the stonework; this just diminished them more. It's probably a good thing it did, because having the operation on each one was the best thing I could have done for myself. They are stronger, and the pain is gone.

My doctor has a sense of humor. He said, "Your hips are like two front tires on a car that have gone flat."

I enjoy all phases of home improvement, especially projects that are a challenge and take me into unknown territories. And, who knows, maybe someday I'll try to fix that toilet or hook up an electrical outlet.

Over time, I have gained more out of life by lessening the fear and believing in myself. I am eager to approach any situation. If I find something way out of my league, I call on my stepson or my contractor or get the information from a home improvement store. And then I try to learn from them.

In the summer of 2006, I ventured outdoors *before* breakfast. This is something I would never attempt in the eighties or nineties. For years, I clung to the fear of past experiences. From swimming every day to frequenting fast food restaurants, I spent too much time going from an indoor environment to an outdoor environment to an indoor environment. Therefore, I resisted as many *ins and outs* as possible. It had always resulted in migraines.

Once I had planted my roots at home, I decided to eliminate going in and out as much as possible, especially first thing in the morning. Living like this eased the pain. But sometimes I was sad as I watched Paul and other people move about in different temperatures any time of the day. They weren't affected. I compared my restrictions to their carefree lifestyle and was jealous at times; however, I still continued in my self-defeating, obsessive safe patterns.

In November 2007, we hired a contractor to install new siding on our home. Because of him and his assistant, I ventured out into the cold more often. Normally, upon leaving the house on a cold, winter day, I moved very quickly toward my car without hesitating in the cold. Ever since my diagnosis of low body temperature, Paul has tried to protect me. He often said I was like the boy in the bubble. As long as I stay protected from the cold and most environmental changes, I could survive. He remembers those days all too well.

In some ways, he wants to protect me too much. Paul's thinking could also hold me back if I let it. I also believe he felt more needed when I depended upon him for everything. Now, I am an independent woman.   At one time, I stayed in this *safe haven* in order to exist and not get sick. It was far less intimidating than trying something new. At one time, if I went outdoors at ten in the morning, or exited the house at all, I was compelled to continue that same obsessive behavior every day. Not anymore. I go out if I have the desire to. The next day is a new day in which I decide how I want to spend it. Every day doesn't have to be an exact repeat performance in order for my life to continue.

The contractor and his assistant came into my life at the ideal time. They often needed my approval on the exterior renovations.

Occasionally, his assistant offered some alternative ideas and suggested a few changes, but the contractor replied, "You need to check with Jill first."

Many times, it would have been easy to tell them I couldn't come out, it was too cold, or I woke up with a migraine. I had accomplished going outdoors in the early morning during the summer; winter was a *different animal.* I knew they needed me. Paul had given me the responsibility of the job, and it was my duty to follow it through.

I convincingly mumbled to myself, "I'll just go out quickly and right back in. Maybe that won't affect me."

Without thinking any further, I changed from a skirt into long pants. Then I added a hat, scarf, and mittens. As I slipped into a pair of boots, my heart began to beat a little faster. Ironically, once I was outdoors, it was crispy, cool, and refreshing. When I returned to the interior of my home, I wasn't overheated from the temperature change. I smiled at myself. And the next time, it was effortless and more natural. It wasn't long before I was ducking out of the house to assess the job, take a few pictures, shovel a little snow, and disperse the rock salt. And I was wearing winter slacks! How cool was that?

My fears had held me back. They were a constant reminder and a reflection of the wreckage in my past. I needed something to help me take that leap of faith and break down barriers. This was a huge modification after thirty years of playing it safe. I strongly believe it wouldn't have happened without my contractor and his assistant.

I had put myself in a cocoon. Most likely, my fears would have kept me within the old lifestyle. For years, Paul and I dictated the schedule, made the rules, and kept everything the same so I wouldn't get sick. In hiring people, not in the family, we had to fit into society and go with the flow. With people we knew, it was easier to make excuses and lean on the old ways, or maybe the timing wasn't right.

This blessing was meant to be so I could move on with my life. The contractor and his assistant were doing God's work. They helped me overcome my fear of being outside in the cold. I was evolving from an entrapment like a butterfly coming out of a cocoon.

This tremendous advancement was another answered prayer. I truly believe all my drastic changes scare Paul. I think he feels he is losing me to that independent woman, which means his job is coming to an end.

Once in awhile, Paul says, "I miss those days in the past. You're never going back there, are you?"

I had refrained from wearing slacks most of my life. How I felt about slacks changed in 2007 when I needed to be protected while outside on a wintry, cold day with my contractor. The more I wore the slacks, the better they felt; I was nice and warm. I never purchased a jacket because it didn't work well with a skirt; my butt and hips and legs were too cold. I started wearing a pair of slacks and a jacket to go grocery shopping and to all doctor appointments. Seems silly to be excited over something so simple, but for me it was a huge achievement and wanted to tell everyone, "Look at me. I'm sixty years old, and I am finally wearing slacks." (I bought my first pair of blue jeans in 2010.)

As a child, I hated long pants. In the winter, for sports or play, I wore them outdoors. Once indoors, I couldn't wait to get them off and away from my skin. I may have had one pair of blue jeans in my teen years, which I never wore.

The one hundred percent polyester had been my trademark for years, and now I was testing out new materials. Paul is pleased I am able to go into a store and find something suitable on the clothing rack — one more necessity I didn't think would ever change. I was sure I would be buried in a wraparound, polyester skirt and top to match.

At least, I am willing to try new fabrics and outfits. My husband always comments on how sexy I look in slacks, so I guess it is also a good reason to wear them.

The need to *control* is still present. This is one of my downfalls. It leads to immense anxiety. It is a common symptom in anorexic nervosa patients. After the first total hip replacement, I was no longer in control. I had to rely on Paul, just like the old days. He totally came through for me as always. Many of the chores I always insisted on doing, he took over and accomplished beautifully. I believe the operation brought us closer together. During the convalescent period, I had to stay somewhat quiet, whether I wanted to or not. My body actually went on vacation, and I had a wonderful rest.

Even with this new lifestyle, which is very positive, I continue to endure the migraines. The difference is I don't wait for the perfect day when I'm feeling my best and the temperature outdoors is to my liking. Whatever calls me outside the house, I do my best to follow it through. If I get a migraine, I tackle it when it happens. At least, I am giving life a chance. I'm on my way to becoming part of the human race.

Most of my self-improvements took place in my home. Going in and out of public buildings is sometimes a problem. I can control the temperatures at home to some degree but not in commercial buildings. In a day-to-day existence, during this time period, you would have found me at home about ninety percent of the time. And even currently, my husband and I do very little socializing. The Internet and the telephone are the largest parts of our social contact. We don't eat in restaurants, go to movies, see stage shows, or take trips that involve overnights. We very rarely have people over for dinner or go to anyone else's home.

I don't accept lunch or dinner dates. If you ask me to meet you for lunch next Tuesday at noon, I can't give you an answer. I don't know until the day arrives. Then, most likely, I'll have a reason to say no. I appreciate the offer. But dining outside my home isn't something I enjoy. I like my home and what it offers, a safe haven, almost free of migraines. I'm past the halfway mark in my life. Whatever time God gives me from now on, I don't want to spend part of it struggling with temperature changes in a restaurant. There was a time in my life when I actually didn't know if I would ever be able to live in a house again without suffering — and maybe a woman, addicted to swimming four times a day, never eating a meal at home. My life is beautiful, and I'm blessed.

I believe when we're addicted or obsessed with a daily pattern, our mind believes in what we're doing because it makes the day easier. We hold on to our behavior with such a tight grip we won't allow ourselves to change and grow and heal. Over time, if we're blessed, we realize how detrimental that addiction has become. Even when someone loves us, like Paul loves me, letting go isn't easy.

My addiction was very deep-rooted and wasn't something I could kick overnight. I also added many other obsessions, which became a security to my survival. It is frightening to give them up, but when released, what a truly beautiful moment in time. We have been given so much in life; life itself is a wondrous gift.

Chapter 30
The Voice of Water

There was a time when water beckoned, and I followed. The water dictated how I led my life. To correct any problem, water became the answer. All through the healing years, water played a big role, a major tool in survival. As I stated earlier, when I couldn't take the torture created from the heat, I ran to water. I finally gave up the swimming. But on a daily basis, I still had to get into some water — no question about it. Even if Paul and I came home late at night, which was rare, I *would not* go to bed without taking a bath.

My migraines normally occurred during the day or at daybreak. The first time I encountered one in the middle of the night, my immediate reaction was a hot bath. Water was the cure for all problems. Usually, my body temperature dropped while lying still. Hot water was a quick way to bring it up. But my first thought was not about my body temperature. I was solely thinking about hiding in the water to fix the pain.

If I was depressed and very agitated or my day wasn't going the way I wanted it or I just didn't feel right, my first thought was to take a hot bath.

There is nothing wrong with using water. My concern was I took it to a destructive level. I couldn't live without it. Water became a drug that took away the agony. Next, it was an obsession; then I had to have it every day, and the simple pleasure was gone.

I wouldn't think of skipping a bath, plus my entire head had to be wet. It just had to be. Every day, I took a bath; I wouldn't consider taking a shower. Water running over me wasn't the same as lying in the water. I needed to be in a horizontal position with the water totally covering me. We even took out our shower, because I was obsessed with only taking a bath. I was sure I would never need a permanent showerhead in the future.

Over time, I realized wetting my head and using a hair dryer gave me more headaches. I decided to bathe every other day. The new routine was acceptable, so I omitted another day and another day until I was down to bathing once a week. Before I knew it, I didn't even want to wet my head once a week. I dreaded washing my hair and even taking a bath.

This new discovery was a relief. I wasn't shackled by another water obsession. Maybe I was dirty and stinky, but I was released from an entrapment. I was amazed at the difference and the freedom it gave me. I had always made myself take a bath or eat a meal exactly the same time of day, every day. When I didn't want to, I still felt I had to stick to the rigid schedule. It didn't matter if I was doing something enjoyable like having sex or watching a movie. I looked at the clock, and whatever I was involved in, it stopped. I'm not sure why. Maybe it gave me security after such an unsettled past. I felt safe with a structured plan — something I could count on and look forward to.

Time and God have been on my side. Little by little, I have eased up on a time schedule. When I'm in an unsettling predicament, there is a little voice in my head that says, "Whatever is happening, there is a reason for it. You may not see it right now, but in time, you will understand."

When I received the prognosis that my two hipbones were shot, it wasn't very good news. My worst fear was leaving Paul alone where he had to do everything himself. I was the main doer in our home. I wasn't sure if he could survive without me. The operation on the first hip was a complete success. Many areas of my life were improved because of the surgery, not just my hip. People were in and out of my room constantly, and there was conversation while I was eating, and I survived. There were no baths, in the hospital, only sponge baths. I wasn't my usual, active self. I was resting in bed. It was a time to relax, sleep, and eat. At home, I probably would have insisted on busying myself with something. So the lifestyle I thought I had to live by was now erased. Ironically, I managed extremely well. Paul took care of everything at home. He picked up where I left off, maybe not exactly the same, but good enough. There was a very strong message in all of this: I could let up on perfection and maybe loosen my schedule a bit. I was at peace and unstressed in the hospital. And I healed very quickly. I realized my life was beginning to be more about *choice*. And getting better was more important than clinging to old ways.

As long as the stitches were in, only sponge baths were allowed. After the surgery, the headaches were almost nonexistent. I connected the two, and I thought maybe taking a sponge bath over a regular bath or shower was helping my migraines. With this assessment, I decided to eliminate a full bath or shower. The days were nearly perfect; I wanted them to continue forever. I didn't take a shower or a bath or wash my hair for three weeks. Most people can't wait to totally soak themselves in water after surgery. I was very happy to exclude it. What was good in the beginning wasn't at the end. Again, a message: because something is excellent one day doesn't mean it will be excellent every day for the rest of my life.

The second operation was, once again, totally successful. The hospital stay was rather unpleasant for many reasons; hence, I was home in three days. I had much more pain but healed quickly. Home therapy was better than outstanding. I recovered much faster than the first time, which makes me wonder if this is how *it was meant to be*.

I don't know about the suffering in the hospital, but those things happen, I guess. I need to mention one incident because it concerns the infamous white hat. During surgery, of course, hats are not allowed. The white hat was given to Paul. After recovery and once I was placed in a room, the plan was for Paul to bring me my white hat. A room wasn't available for quite some time. Paul wasn't able to wait; daylight diminished into darkness, and he also felt the cats needed to be fed. When I opened my eyes, the new hip was fine. Unfortunately, the room was freezing, and my head was void of a hat. This is something I make sure never happens. The staff even had jackets on. The nurses put blankets on my head; for me it wasn't the same as a hat. My head continued to throb with pain. From this point forward, everything else seemed to go wrong. I was relieved of a considerable amount of agonizing stress when it was time to go home.

This hip surgery occurred eighteen months after the first one. Again, I was blessed to receive more than the new hip. God brought a young woman into my life. She had lived in the neighborhood for about twenty years. The only time we engaged in conversation was on warm, summer days. We chatted briefly if she happened to be taking a walk past my house or if I walked by her home. She knew about my surgery, and after I came home, she offered to help me with the bathing.

Every morning, she arrived promptly at ten o'clock. She had a wonderful sense of humor. I found myself laughing every day we were together; her infectious laugh greatly improved my health. As a conclusion to each sponge bath, she massaged my legs with divine cranberry butter cream lotion. I felt as if I had my own health spa at home. She was amazing. I truly believe her magical hands hastened the healing.

This time, as soon as the stitches came out, I was in the shower! After hip surgery, a shower is easier than a bath until the hip is totally healed. I wasn't too keen on that either. I didn't like showers. As soon as possible, I would be back to taking baths. Psychologically, I believed a bath adjusted and improved the temperature of my body. The water encased my body versus running over it. Then, when I stepped out into the air, I was able to better cope with whatever temperatures were around me. This was not a scientific conclusion, but my own assumption.

Ever since 1981, or thereabouts, I had to lie down on my bed before and after a bath. The need to lie down was more than an *on-and-off* habit. There weren't days when I skipped lying down. Before *every* bath this obsession was eminent. I would not get into the bathtub until I quieted my body enough to feel cool. Then I accepted a hot bath.

I was very much at ease when I was with my new friend, and the old obsession never entered my mind. I'm not sure why it was so easy with her at my side. And alone, I couldn't bring myself to change this obsessive-compulsive behavior. Maybe because we laughed so much, it washed away my fears. God placed her here for a reason. When it was time for a shower, she and I were either deep in discussion or were laughing; therefore, I just undressed and stepped into the shower. My friend was an instrument in the transformation of letting this obsession go.

A short time ago, I thought I was free by not bathing at all; that wasn't freedom. I didn't see it at the time, but it was just another fear. By totally omitting a bath to evade something else, the problem wasn't corrected.

This wonderful gal probably had no idea what she had accomplished. She took part in one of the most important changes in my life! After the shower, she and I sat and talked while she put the lotion on my legs. During these minutes, I naturally cooled down. This is where lying on the bed came in. I didn't need to lie down anymore; this quiet time did the trick. After we finished, she went home, and I continued with my day.

As I watched her, I could see she was rather warm and uncomfortable. The more we talked the more I learned. My friend didn't do well in warm temperatures! Our tiny bathroom is on the top floor over the furnace, therefore, the warmest room in the house. The heat created by the running water plus being somewhat active — I believe most anyone would be drenched in sweat. She never complained. She never missed a day for three weeks. I am forever grateful for her genuine kindness and for giving up her comfort zone for mine.

One morning, my friend wasn't on schedule. I paced. Every few minutes, I glanced at the grandfather clock. Usually, the shower was at ten o'clock, and I ate lunch at eleven o'clock. When she arrived, we went through our usual, daily routine. The worry was for nothing. I realized I could choose my time to shower and eat my meals.

Occasionally, some of my changes aren't long lasting. I never know until the change settles within my soul, and I'm comfortable with it. After several weeks, I knew this shift was permanent. When I think of this gift, I close my eyes and smile. The angels must be singing with me as I experience this beautiful freedom. This liberty has not been enjoyed for over thirty years.

Before November 26, 2008, my bathing schedule was carved in stone. I made myself follow it out of fear. The longer I let go of the restrictions, the less I thought about the time. I now shower whenever I please — no set time. After being set free, I can't imagine being told I have to take a shower or bath at the exact same time daily with no choice or flexibility.

I believe God prepared me for this moment; I was finally ready. This wonderful element in my new life has spun off into many more wonderful freedoms. Sometimes I can't believe it really happened. It made me feel exceedingly good about myself. Left to my own devices, it may not have happened. I was blessed by a genuine, sincere, and kind woman with a huge heart who came my way and spent so much quality time with me. Because of her, the changes were much easier. And from these days together, we have become the best of friends.

Coming off the drugs after the first surgery was very difficult, especially being an addict. I was ill with migraines for five days. I was good at comparing. After the second surgery, I feared the same. I allowed this worry to mount up. I had lived a life of patterns and repetition. This was a normal reaction for me. And *lo and behold*, I didn't get sick. I developed a few migraines, but I was able to manage the pain with a drug that could be taken long term, thus, safer.

Over the years, most drugs had bad side affects. Bed rest was the only option until the horrible pain ended. This drug was different. I was given some relief. I was optimistic and anticipated more pain-free days. Thinking happy thoughts, and practicing biofeedback, in combination with the drug, I was able to function enough to stay out of bed. And pleasant conversations with Paul directed my thoughts toward *positive instead of negative*.

This was definitely another life lesson. No two events will be identical. I assumed that both hip surgeries would be about the same — not true at all. Everything I experience will have its own dimension.

I don't think I ever truly realized how suffocating an obsession would become. And how afraid it would be to give it up. But on the flip side, for me I don't believe all my obsessions or habits were totally bad. As long as I recognized them and eventually was able to let go and learn from them. The professionals may differ with me. But in my opinion, seeing a therapist and being told to stop an obsession or addiction within a given time isn't always the best advice. That did not work at all in my situation. For me, it was timing, faith, and the people who came across my path.

Sometimes, without even knowing it is happening, I let go of ironclad, compulsive, habitual behavior. Then I experienced an awakening. I realized how much better my life was and wonder why I didn't change sooner. My advice is: don't beat yourself up if you have some behavior patterns that are a little unorthodox. When the time is right, and you are ready to *kick* them out of your life, they will disappear.

At times, the water relates to an unpleasant past. It's a place I don't want to return to. I'm learning to enjoy water for the moment I am in it. I am not desperate to feel it around my body or use it to move to the next part of my day. I will survive. Depending on water to get through the day is a thought I don't ever want again.

In 2007, while writing this book, I again decided to see how long I could delay taking a bath. After recovering from a migraine, the pain stopped; a tremendous relief; I wanted to hold on to the comfortable feeling. I decided to eliminate all bathing or any other habit. It was nice to be stripped of all dependencies and just work with what God gave me: myself. No fans, no air-conditioning, no hot, no cold, no water, no colas, no coffee, no drugs, no one particular food all the time, and even no makeup. I thought of it as the raw me, living my life without using anything else as an aid. It proved to be very joyful and productive.

I remained in the house for about a week with no outdoor temperature changes. I ate healthy and abstained from Coke — I have found Coke to help with migraines, although too much can boot me in the butt and make them worse! It was like a fast from daily habits. I felt like I had a fresh start. I thought I wanted *rawness* to last forever, but it could develop into living in a bubble again. I've come too far to stop progress now. I have to admit a bath felt very good after abstaining!

I keep reminding myself it is important to venture on and go outside the box once again. I gain some and lose some. It always amazes me how taking chances and trying something new is rewarding, uplifting, and a learning experience. Whatever direction my journey takes me now, I know in my heart God is with me; and with Him, anything is possible. I believe there are only good things to come in my healing.

Chapter 31
The Caregiver

I truly thought God had outdone himself with all the blessings he bestowed upon me. I was very satisfied with how my life was going. What happened to Paul wasn't a blessing, but it did lead to an enormous breakthrough for me, which, in turn, benefited us both.

It was March 2009. Paul's body was slowing down, and he didn't act right. I knew God was giving me a sign. As it turned out, Paul had bronchitis and sleep apnea; therefore, his activities lessened. He became disoriented; his words were slurred; he fell asleep whenever he sat at the table, even during a conversation; his breathing was terrible, and I was scared. A trip to the ER followed, but he was released. His condition worsened, and he was admitted with pneumonia.

The hospital environment and I didn't blend well together. It was way too cool in his room. I stayed at home taking care of the household duties, the cats and my health. He was fine with that. In fact, he insisted.

After being released, Paul continued to do the grocery shopping; however, that was becoming more and more difficult. I saw him huffing and puffing as he carried the groceries into the house. One trip and he had to sit down and rest. I didn't always see him when he returned, and I'd find ice cream sitting in the sun, because he didn't have the energy to carry it any further.

His falling asleep throughout the day continued, so I scheduled a sleep apnea test. In the meantime, there was a possibility he could fall asleep at the wheel. One day he dozed off for ninety minutes, while sitting in his car in our driveway. I parked my car behind his. Paul was not able to drive until his "nodding off" was under control. I then knew we had to make some changes.

Although I didn't know it, because of my recent improvements I was ready to take on more responsibilities. With Paul's car parked, it was perfect timing. I attempted to do all the errands outside the house. I had a little difficulty with the temperatures, but I managed. I decided to go only once a week and hit as many stores as possible all in one day.

Over the years, Paul even filled up the cars with gas, so I didn't have to stand out in the cold. If we wanted to rent a movie, he went to the video store. He saw how I suffered from the drastic temperature changes. After he took sick in March, I became the errand lady. And, for the most part, I enjoyed it. At first, I suffered a little from all the "ins and outs," but in time, I created a system. Before I knew it, shopping was like taking a shower; I just did it. My favorite radio station, which played the oldies, was a great way to start the *to do* list. One morning, as I was parking my car at the bank, "Morning Train" was playing. I sat in the car with my eyes closed and sang along, until the song ended — the joys of growing older!

I scheduled Paul for a sleep apnea test in May. The doctor wanted him in their building at 6:45 p.m. I was okay with that. The next morning, Paul was to be picked up before 7:00 a.m. I was a little nervous about me going out of the house at an early hour and on a cool morning, but I told Paul one way or another, he would get home.

The following morning, I was up at 5:30 fed the cats, ate breakfast, dressed, and was on the highway at 6:30. The sun was just coming up, the air was crisp and great to breathe, there were very few cars on the highway, and it was so quiet. The morning was gorgeous. I was close to tears as my inner emotion swelled up inside of me.

I murmured to myself, "This is a beautiful way to start the day, and dear, Lord, thank you for allowing me to bathe in this moment."

The eye doctor found cataracts in Paul's eyes. Surgery was scheduled along with many appointments. The time of day wasn't the best: 7:40 a.m., 9:30 a.m., and an emergency call at the doctor's office at 9:15 p.m.

There were other appointments that fell on nice sunny days when I anticipated working in the garden. Appointments for myself were never scheduled this early in the morning. It would be an interference with my routine. And I feared the uneven temperatures. I attempted to keep my skin protected from outside temperatures until after lunch. Once lunch was finished I was able to venture out. There was always the fear of a migraine. I set myself up for failure before it happened.

When Paul needed me I had to become the caregiver.

Several times Paul said, "I can drive myself. I can walk. Drop me off, and I'll get home on my own."

I knew this option was out of the question. When I first started taking Paul to his appointments in March, the weather was on the cool side. The indoor temperatures were moderate, and I managed quite well. As the season changed the indoor temperature became more difficult. Paul continually told me to go home and come back, which I finally did. During the warmer months, I cannot tolerate AC set lower than seventy-nine degrees. If I attempt to wear more clothing, all I do is perspire, my skin feels clammy, and a headache develops. Paul used to kid me and say, "If I could find a space suit, I'd buy it for you. Then you could control the temperature around you."

Maybe I'm not supposed to control all the temperatures. I do that in my own home as much as possible. I am challenged when I leave my house. I do the best I can; I know one way or another I will survive.

We decided it was time to take Paul's car off the road. I can only imagine how difficult this is for any senior citizen. Even though Paul does enjoy staying at home, he was a little hesitant. He didn't want to feel trapped. Surprisingly, he was satisfied with the quietness of our home and being with our cats and me, although I probably drive him crazy sometimes.

Many household chores were becoming difficult for Paul. His breathing was heavy, and he had gained a considerable amount of weight. And his knees hurt. I began taking care of everything inside and outside of our home. From the garden to the grocery run, doctor appointments, gas station, prescription pickup, some snow removal, and anything else we needed. I thought I had it altogether and was conquering my new role. My days were so full I didn't even think about getting into a project to stay busy. I was plenty active with no time for much else!

I thought I was appreciative when Paul was doing all the grocery shopping and the errands outside the house. When I took on the role, I could truly see his full-time job. He conquered it all and never complained.

From March to May of 2009 I was able to conduct the daily activities without a migraine forcing me to go to bed. Then all of a sudden, I had a week of more headaches than normal. One morning the pain would not go away. I took a pill, and still the pain grew worse. I knew what was next. I had trouble walking, nausea overwhelmed me, and soon I had my head over the toilet bowl. I was able to prepare three meals for Paul and feed the cats. The in-between time was spent in bed in agonizing pain. My beautiful Duma sensed I was in trouble, probably from all the moaning he heard. His furry warm body, snuggled close to my hip, as I lay in bed waiting for the pain to cease. When I ran to the toilet, he followed. Wherever I was, Duma was with me. These episodes take their toll and "knock me for a loop." Once the pain leaves, my senses come alive. Everything smells wonderful, food tastes unbelievably good, and my brain is rested and more alert. The day is beautiful and all is right with the world.

As Paul's caregiver in 2009, I repeatedly accepted unfavorable temperatures within a closer time frame. I became stronger mentally and physically. I could overcome just about anything. I only had two severe migraines within eight months — an enormous improvement. And I fulfilled more of my responsibilities.

One of the migraines was much worse than usual. I had pushed my body past its limit without realizing it. I was overtired. My mind was in the right place; my body wasn't able to keep up. I went into seclusion. I pulled back into my cocoon. I cancelled any upcoming appointments within the week. The even temperatures inside my home led to peace and contentment, and that was better than suffering.

During this interlude, Paul was scheduled for a colonoscopy. I could not drive him to the hospital. I was not ready for the pain to return, not after the horrific migraine I had just undergone. I gave in and called his daughter. I felt as if I had failed. I wasn't carrying out the duties I claimed I could handle. Once again, I was depending on someone else.

I continued to stay in the house for over a week. Then I realized I wasn't living. I was playing life safe again. I concluded that during a major healing process, it is good to take it slow. I tend to rush into new challenges with gusto. Maybe I took on too much, too fast. I was being given a lesson: slow down and try again, and this time put the speed on low.

Temperature changes drastically affect my ability to function properly. It truly appears I am environmentally challenged. Most people probably function quite nicely *outdoors* in a seventy-degree temperature; I try; I suffer. That's all there is to it. On a nice sunny day, with the temperature at a pleasant seventy degrees, I open a window to water my flower boxes. The air hits my face; I have a sharp pain in my head and an immediate ice-pick headache, plus my body perspires a clammy cool sweat. Doing all I do within the vicinity of my home is one thing. I am able to bounce back most of the time. I protect my body by incorporating my own comfort zone. And I exercise. That elevates my body temperature, and eventually the headache disappears. To participate in anything where I have to drive over an hour away from my house is questionable. I have found that during our enjoyable outings, most of the time is spent sitting, which allows my body to cool much more than it ought to. The desire to be involved is there; however, cause and effect continues to linger in my mind.

If my body changes, it does. If it doesn't, I'll deal with it the best I can. I have been coping for years, and God's rewards have been many.

I tell myself, "Thinking about a situation that hasn't occurred isn't going to give me the answers now. I'll cope with the situation when it happens."

As I grow older, healthier and wiser, I realize that I can barely control my own life. I certainly have no control over how long it will last;

therefore, it is important to savor what I have. Why waste time worrying about what "average Joe" might be thinking. Nor do I feel guilty about not participating in events or activities that cause me great discomfort. Isn't it said, "Why should you not judge a man until you have walked a mile in his shoes?" I am blessed. Many people have tried my shoes on; they have attempted to walk with me.

Writing this book was one of the most wonderful gifts I could have given myself. The dedication wiped away most of my obsessions. I probably haven't been able to sit this long since I was in college. I think it's safe to say I've been in motion for over forty years, from the swimming addiction to every other obsession along the way. For years, I didn't indulge in an activity that quieted my body for any length of time. My days did not leave any free time for such things as creative writing. Telling my story in book form allowed this to happen. I was also able to stop whatever I was doing in order to jot down a thought or write a paragraph: in the middle of a meal, during the night or after a shower, and even before I was dry. I just had to get my brainstorm on paper.

Before I started writing this book, I was complaining to a doctor, "I can't gain weight." She told me all I had to do was sit more. And she was right!

Writing allowed me to become lost in the words and forget everything else. Time meant nothing. The weeks flew by; I could have easily enjoyed a few more hours in the day. I'd like my life to slow up a bit. It would be nice to remain at my present age for about ten or twenty years!

On the cool unpleasant days Paul performed the simple outside tasks. For example he fed the birds, emptied the trash, picked up the mail, or fed any stray cat passing by the house. And because he had for so long, I let him continue. In the spring of 2009, our roles were reversed. It was necessary for me to take care of *all* the chores when Paul was sick. Now it comes naturally. I am almost over the bridge from the *fear of* — to — *I can do it*. (The only time I hold back is during and after an intense migraine.)

Paul sometimes asks in the afternoon when dinner will be ready and what are we having? I don't have a clue. We eat when I place the meal on the table. Before my second hip surgery, and my friend's companionship, I forced myself to suffer unnecessarily, because I was afraid to change.

I insisted on taking a bath daily at nine or ten o'clock. After gardening I was sweaty, hot, and dirty. The schedule never wavered. I didn't allow myself to step out of my obsessive behavior. I now shower whenever I can fit it in to my day or when I need to be clean. And I even skip a day.

I go to the grocery store early in the morning, come home and have lunch, and then go to another store. Praise God.

I am able to step outside the house whenever I please. People can stop in to see us anytime. I am able to leave a meal, go outdoors, and come back in and finish eating. Whenever Paul or my cats need me, I'm available. There are no restrictions to the hour of the day. The entire day is open to chance, for whatever may come along. I may prefer some of it at certain times, but I can adapt to *almost* anything within the circumference of my home. I say *almost*, because I still have a few more challenges. And stress is one of them. My body isn't always willing to keep up the pace. I try not to dwell on it. It is what it is. Hopefully, in time I will become a stronger woman.

The challenges have been many. I believe the advancement has put me in a position to accomplish *almost* anything I set my mind to.

I mentioned to a girlfriend that I'm a normal housewife. I have no time. I'm running in all directions. The response was, when someone we love is ill or desperately needs us, it is amazing how we can step up to the plate and do more than we thought possible.

This is probably very true; however, I didn't even think of it in the same way. I can do the work physically, and I am the first to step up and take charge. The migraines tear my down.

When I was seventeen and a senior in high school, our class traveled to Washington, DC. The bus only made minimal restroom stops. When they occurred, the group was told how time much was allowed. This particular stop was a "quickie." I had to empty my bladder, and because I didn't have enough time, I wasn't able to urinate. I held my bladder from upstate New York all the way to Washington, DC. From that moment on, I was afraid the same thing would happen when I had to empty my bladder. Every train ride into New York City, when I worked for McCall's Pattern Company, I feared the same scenario. One restroom, heaven forbid someone was waiting in the lounge to use the toilet. I mentioned earlier in my story of a train trip to Florida. It took a couple of days. I wasn't able to empty my bladder during the entire trip.

To this day, when I'm admitted into the hospital I am unable to use a bedpan. When I first moved into Paul's house, I used to lock the bathroom door and stay in there for hours. I couldn't urinate. The surroundings were new, other roomers moving about, and I was afraid someone was waiting to use the toilet. At the time, he knew nothing of my past. He threatened to take the locks off the door, because it was so unusual for someone to sit on the toilet for so long. Often doctors need urine samples. I have had to remake appointments because I wasn't able to put even one drop in a cup.

Even after all these years I cannot urinate if Paul is in the room, unless he is in the shower with the curtain closed. (And only recently has that advancement happened.) Because we are soul mates, he has allowed me to work through my issues at my own pace and, hopefully, someday conquer them all.

Another, but similar, situation came about through choice. When I lived in New York City and conquered the feat of losing weight, I restricted my diet to such an extent for six days that my bowels didn't work properly. The diet was a nationally recognized diet at the time. It appeared to be extremely healthy. I still think it is. The food groups were covered, and the variety of fruits and vegetables were excellent. I walked whenever possible. I ate very small portions. I eliminated all fats, pasta, potatoes and rice. Only after I binged and took a laxative on the seventh day did I have a bowel movement. This went on for months and months; being thin was more important than thinking about my health. It's a wonder I stayed alive.

I mention these last circumstances only as an example to show how easy it is to acquire fears, phobias, habits, or whatever labels anyone wants to use. In the end, fears seem to defeat the human soul. The heat I felt, that is still uncertain as to how it all began. Right now, it doesn't matter. I'm a survivor.

I've heard people say, "If I only had this much knowledge when I was a teenager." I wonder if we really would live our lives any differently. I think it takes years to learn about our limitations and our behavior, good or bad. As we grow, hopefully, it becomes a positive part of who we are. As seniors, I believe we are given a gift from God; we become more aware. Growing old can be a beautiful experience. It all depends on how we view it. Can our destiny be changed? Who knows if that is possible. But we can come to our senses and start to take care of our body, appreciate our blessings, and love one another and ourselves.

I had accepted my limitations/obsessions as ordinary for me, never thinking that my lifestyle would change. And if I was able to change, I didn't think it would last more than a few days, and then I'd be back to my old ways.

When Paul became ill in 2009, there was a voice telling me to go forth and walk the walk; I'd be fine. Don't think about it. Just do it; you are ready.

One of my doctors sent me a wonderful note. In it, she quoted, "Necessity is the teacher of good coping [survival] skills." And she added, "Thanks, Paul, for giving Jill the rope. She really is capable and strong."

Chapter 32
Change, through God,
Brought Me to the Good Life

My journey thus far has been from 1972 to 2009. All the changes that took place along the way were not easy. I don't think I ever made the changes without outside motivation. I was not an easy person to change. My body dictated most of them; I believe God intervened many times. Each change gave me a brighter tomorrow, even though, at the time, I didn't think it would. Often, I fought the change. I believed my ways were a level of perfection. I was in control, and my obsessions worked for me.

Finally, I am beginning to let go of demanding perfection from myself. I am aiming toward becoming better. When all is said and done, the changes are positive and good. I have had many *a-ha* moments intertwined with the less fortunate ones.

Sitting still has always been a challenge. Thanks to God, it began to improve. Over the years, I craved being in motion. Whether the trait stemmed from the compulsion to swim, due to the overwhelming warmth I felt, I'm not sure. Whenever I sat to read a book, I lasted about twenty minutes. Paul and I were able to watch television for approximately sixty minutes. Whenever I was very active throughout the day, I rarely took a break. On those evenings, once in a blue moon, I'd watch television for two hours. When I was in a doctor's waiting room, I spend most of the time pacing up and down the hall until my name is called. I often walked out. I have this overwhelming urge to move my body. Then when I was confined in unfavorable room temperatures, it felt as if someone placed a tight rubber band around my head, which created a sharp pain on the right side of my brain and worked its way to my eyes, cheek, and jaw bone. Appointments were not something I relished.

Whenever Paul and I went shopping, Paul stood in line for me. The forced air overhead contributed to an immediate headache. Therefore, I waited in another part of the store or in the car. As time went on, Paul did all the grocery shopping; I stayed at home.

With each new change, what I thought *had to be* slowly started to disappear. After several years, I decided it was time to attempt the grocery shopping on my own. The checkout area was usually better than in the past.

My biggest downfall was the dairy section being unbelievably cold. A friend suggested I go to customer service and explain my plight. She said to tell them I get migraine headaches from the cold and could someone go to the dairy section for me. The store was very accommodating.

Telephone conversation is a wonderful way to stay connected to family and friends. However, heat still builds up in my head and creates pressure. After switching the phone from ear to ear, then holding it away from my head, I start pacing up and down the room. Walking releases the tension, and the heat. It becomes a nice tool. If anyone finds himself or herself pacing, you are not alone!

In portions of my book, I talk about being bothered by cold and moving air. In another paragraph, I mention that becoming too warm is difficult. Both are true. Any environmental change takes a toll on my body. In the past, I went in the wrong direction to fix how I felt. I am finally confident in the choices I make to improve my illness.

Obstacles still occur almost daily, but they challenge me to overcome. If I succeed, I shed just another layer of an obsession or addiction. It isn't water anymore. Most of the time, it is fear — the fear of being where it is too hot or too cold, how my body will react to the elements, and how I will cope with it. Given all this time, I now have insight into my inner makeup. I am aware of what I can and cannot do in my daily walk, just like any other illness. I dress properly for different temperatures. Through trial and error, I know what to eat to keep my weight and body temperature where it should be for a healthy life.

From my own perspective, I believe I have the right to say when something happens out of the ordinary or when an unplanned event materializes or when a challenge arises; those times are the best days.

I now know I can cool myself off from the food I eat, by lying down, doing biofeedback, meditating, casual walking, and doing tai chi. Thinking happy positive thoughts and engaging in pleasant conversation also helps. I don't need to freeze myself or immerse my body in cold water in order to put food in my mouth and get through the day.

Maybe some people will wonder why I couldn't have done all these things a long time ago. It has taken years to get where I am today. The addiction had to be shrunk little by little over time — and in my own time. It was also a learning experience.

As the years went by, and my mind was able to concentrate on other things besides swimming and cold water, I was able to observe and learn about my body and surroundings.

I read an article about energy. It is all around us. Too much energy can affect people in different ways. At times, I need to be alone when I eat. This is so I don't drown in warmth and lose my appetite. By being alone, I am able to keep myself at a more constant temperature. It quiets my body, and I can consume more food. At first, I didn't know why this was true; I thought it was a phobia. After reading this article, I came to the conclusion that people around me were creating extra energy. The extra energy then produces a heat, which I absorb.

This also happens when I'm with friends, having a wonderful time talking and laughing. In the beginning, I am fine; but as the energy increases with more and more laughing, I get too warm, and my face turns red. Sometimes, I get a migraine. The same principle is happening. Even a good thing like laughing creates more energy than my body can handle. This doesn't mean I don't like to laugh. It means I know what is happening to me and why. I don't have to run away from it; I have learned how to compensate for it.

I have other ways to balance my challenges. I never end a meal with anything cold. Cold lowers my body temperature and gives me a headache. If I eat something cold, it is alternated with a hot item. Even cold fruit isn't eaten cold. I dunk it into hot tea, so it becomes a moderate temperature. These little peculiarities have helped a great deal. They make life a little more manageable. I believe if a simple, weird act can prevent a very bad migraine, it seems ridiculous not to do it, whether other people watching think it odd or not.

From the time Paul and I ordered a pizza on an impulse, I have incorporated more foods into my diet. Years ago, I played it safe by staying with the same foods. For a very long time, I wouldn't indulge in cake, pie, candy, or ice cream. I was afraid they would make me so warm I couldn't stay indoors; therefore, I avoided them.

While I am cooking, I never taste a recipe. I avoid snacking in between meals altogether. The fear of an altered human state still lingers within my thoughts. I still don't trust my body completely. It is safer to just stick to mealtime. Then I have the assurance of counteracting with another food, in case my body is uncomfortable.

I have finally come to a place where I am comfortable eating most anything I desire, in moderation (at mealtime). I am able to eat my cake or a piece of homemade, dark chocolate or my homemade granola without eating the entire container. The urge to binge is gone. A small amount now is satisfying, as long as I mix it with one or more low-heat foods, which would be fruit and water. My body seems to tell me when I need a treat.

At one time, I was afraid to buy a new oven. Our old, gas stove had the knobs on the front. I placed my kitchen chair so I could lean over to turn them on or off when needed; I used the gas jets for extra heat in the room. Being close, I didn't have to stand and walk to the stove. The movement of walking heated me up, and I never finished my food. Once I sat down to eat, I didn't get up until the end of the meal.

One minute, I'm stating I need heat, and in the very next sentence, I'm talking about being too warm. This was a catch-22 dilemma. When I was at rest, I cooled too much, and any movement heated me up — simple as that.

My *furry kids* changed me. I believe my cats were sent to me at the most opportune time. I was ready to accept another challenge. My two youngest felines were born on our patio. Their mama abandoned them. From the day the kittens were born, they didn't have a mother to tend to their needs. I had to be her. God knew it was time for me to take on a new challenge. When the kittens required my attention, I couldn't ignore them. It didn't matter if I was eating, or they wanted to be held at one o'clock in the morning. I had to be there for them. Our older cats vomit at the most inopportune time. I felt it was my responsibility to clean it up — not in an hour, but right when it happened.

When my arthritis flares up I prefer to sit; however, when I'm needed, the up-and-down movement is good exercise. The healthier I become, the more demands there are. I believe I'm being tested. When I am in the middle of a meal, I am finally able to get up and move around to any area of the house, then return to the meal like nothing out of the ordinary has happened. I believe this more and more: circumstances happen for a reason. I am growing in leaps and bounds. I am blessed and fulfilled, because the healing process is moving at a much faster speed.

Situations can tear people apart and bring them back together stronger than ever. Sometimes, I feel sad because a big portion of my existence was spent being ill and addicted. Even so, it has brought me to a place in my life where I believe it is more special, because I lived through an addiction. I love my family and friends; they complete me and give the days more meaning and joy.

On my road to recovery, I jumped many hurdles each year, but the past nine years have been the most significant. Each transformation becomes less fearful. I feel secure with my advancement because I'm growing stronger in knowing who I am. It is exciting to see I don't need the set patterns I once did. I realize it is healthier to be spontaneous and take each day as it comes. Before, when told to take a chance on change, for me, it was out of the question. I was fortunate to have a man who let me take my own time to heal and to figure out what my needs were. With God and my husband's love, I am getting there.

Ever since 1993, Paul and I have eaten breakfast and dinner together. I have tried including him in all four meals. However, I prefer just the two.

Over the years, eating has always been a big issue. It isn't that I don't like to eat; I promised myself a long time ago I would only eat under favorable conditions, and I'm not able to let go of my thinking on the subject. Mealtime would have a happy atmosphere. It would be a positive experience. I have found that when I'm happy, at peace, and relaxed, I consume more food. I enjoy what I am eating. I feel pleased with what I've chosen to eat and the quantity I consume. I leave the table satisfied with my brain mentality elevated, which all leads to a more productive life.

This evaluation comes after years of frustrating surroundings and an unbalanced lifestyle where barely survived my own chaos. Over the years, I struggled with adverse conditions while attempting to eat a meal. I made a pledge to myself; if and when I found serenity and was able to finally sit down and eat a meal, no one would ever take that sanctity away from me. This sounds truly idyllic and probably more like a fairy tale existence, but having a history of anorexia nervosa, I vowed this promise to myself.

There are always times when conversation isn't pleasant. News is talked about in most households, of which most is depressing. There are oodles of other negative topics. I just choose not to hear them while I'm eating. Most of the time, our conversations are wonderful, but sometimes the other *stuff* creeps in.

I find lunchtime is the most difficult for some reason. I choose to be alone and, hopefully, to have some peace and quiet. At the end of the day, when I've about had it and need a bit of *unraveling time*, I enjoy having a snack in silence by myself, except for my cats; they don't talk much.

Paul accepts all of this and tries to understand. When I need to remind him of these *alone* times, he cheerfully complies. I thoroughly enjoy eating breakfast and dinner with my husband. The other two meals will change in time at my own pace. I know it will happen someday.

This new life with new changes has given me the existence I only dreamed about. With this exuberance, I still get horrible migraines, mostly from environmental, temperature changes. I have tried numerous drugs and very little work. I attempt to not let the migraines interrupt my life. Any migraine sufferer knows the pain they inflict; it is indescribable.

Trying to find a miracle drug is difficult. One works; then it doesn't. Trial and error appears to be the pattern. As I said before, I'm not much on staying with a drug if it doesn't work. I'd rather not use any. When I am headache free, not only is the pain gone but also, the psychological effect is great. Knowing I'm not dependent on anything is wonderful and gives me a fuller life.

The most successful migraine treatment was an opiate drug I received while I was in the hospital for my hip surgery. In my case, this type of medication cannot be taken long term. It was my understanding that the drug was highly addictive and only to be used post surgery for a specific amount of time. Because this medicine proved so successful for my migraines, I found it tough to terminate; the relief I received was remarkable. Out of all my complaints, severe migraines top the list, although body temperature can never be dismissed as unimportant along with my eating habits and body weight.

The Fioricet works and then it doesn't; I never know. It also must be used sparingly. Overuse defeats its purpose. At the first sign of a headache, it becomes too easy to pop a pill in my mouth; and before long, I need too many. The less I consume, the better.

The majority of the time, I deal with them as best I can through alternative medicine or ways of relaxation. When all else fails, I still have to go to bed. The end result hasn't changed. What is different? My mind-set is. The migraines don't happen every day, so during the headache-free moments, I don't dwell on the *what if*, I get a headache, syndrome; I carry on as if I never get them.

I often overtax my body and don't listen to my inner voice saying, "Okay, you've had enough for today." It's an obsession; only this time, it isn't cold water. My excuse: It's good to be living again and to lose myself in another world — a world of being creative and productive. I see this as a positive result, plus it feels good, and I'm enjoying it.

I am not totally healed. I still have work to do. I tend to obsess, which can also lead to an addiction. I have never been one to do things in moderation. Whatever I take on, I do it to excess and then some. As a teen, when I learned to water ski, I wanted to ski every day. In the winter, I went skating and snow skiing as much as possible. That sounds good, but I went even when I was exhausted. I broke my leg because of my thought patterns.

I have been told that once I am on a roll, no one can stop me — like painting every room in the house or buying plants when I don't need them. I continually look for projects, which, in turn, creates more work. When I've had enough for the day, I just have to do a little more until I'm so tired I don't eat or sleep enough. Sometimes, I think I treat every project as if I were employed. I have my undertaking to look forward to, and to work at, the same as working for a company. I become a workaholic.

I know being obsessed is harmful, yet I keep doing it to myself. I have come a long way from a cold-water addiction, but I have taken on some other needs to replace it. I strongly believe I've made great progress, for the obvious reasons, and I finally recognize my obsessive-compulsive behavior.

I have an amazing man who has stuck by me through everything. He is supportive of everything I do. Paul overflows with an amazing amount of unconditional love; believe me, he is tested every day. I couldn't expect anything more from him. He does everything humanly possible to make me happy. I often tell him he doesn't get enough out of this relationship for himself.

Paul always says, "If you are happy, then I am happy. That is the only gift I need out of life."

He has been my biggest fan since the first day we met. He is the love of my life. He saved my life.

One time, when we were talking, Paul said, "When you were struggling all those years, you didn't have any joy in your life, did you?"

I told him that isn't true. Once the day was about over, around nine in the evening, then my day started. I enjoyed the music and dance. I enjoyed the few friends I had. At one time, swimming was my total joy. The entire cold-water obsession — the whole routine of swimming and showers every day plus the involved preparation before eating a meal — was not joyful. I knew I wanted to stay alive. Maybe that was all my brain needed to keep me going.

I feel it is never too late to improve, to heal, or to move forward — and become the person I want to be or make better the person I am. So what, if it takes my lifetime? I believe, with each new awakening, I feel more blessed with my existence. I thank God I am alive. There are times when I sit quietly, and then I get a chill. At that exact moment, my brain puts a stop to the electronic world I live in and the *to do* list I have created.

A flashing thought interrupts everything else. I say to myself, "Someday, I will not be sitting here. I will leave this world forever." At this instant, I realize how precious my life is. All the craziness of the day, and what seems to be important, really isn't.

I am very content as I sit in my home, looking out the kitchen window. I am happy to be living my life with a fantastic man and my precious cats. At this very minute, I'm experiencing a different level of existence. It is a meditative state of mind, where the real joy comes from watching the clouds in the sky, the sun shining on a stray cat, a beautiful red bird trying to balance himself as the wind blows the tree branch, or the rain dribbling down a window pane.

I find peace within from this picture, not from a materialistic item I purchased. At least, for a moment, I realize I am okay. Even the squirrel that I normally consider a nuisance, because he eats up all the birdseed, isn't annoying at this particular time. Sitting still for more than ten minutes and doing absolutely nothing takes practice and patience — what a peaceful reward and wonderful habit. For many years, those elements were not a part of my life.

What tomorrow will bring, no one knows. The future for me looks much brighter as each day evolves. A huge amount of weight has been lifted off my back, and I can breathe a lot easier. I know there will always be room for improvement, but the life I have now is one hundred percent better than what I had many, long years ago.

The journey to heal has brought me to a very good place in my life. I believe, with an addiction, one needs to think about taking small steps and recognize the victory in each. That way, the unsettling lifestyle isn't so overwhelming and discouraging. On most days, I am very rewarded by God's blessing. I don't think life is meant to be perfect. I believe I became stronger with challenges.

God has blessed me in so many ways. I prayed to Him daily for a life in warmth rather than in cold. I asked for assistance with living a more normal, acceptable life. He answered my prayers.

I hope my journey is long, and thus far, it has given a lost life back to me. I have been provided with this book to write and share with my readers. I hope I have touched some hearts, healed some hearts, and given hope to those struggling with addictions. There is life after an addiction.

Please, keep the faith and never give up on anything you attempt to achieve. A day is only one day of your life. The tomorrows can always be better.

In peace, there is love.
in both, there is serenity and eternity.

Afterword

In 2010 I believed my life was almost where I wanted it to be. Even though there were more improvements to be made, I believe time and God will heal all. I still fall short once in awhile and wonder where my strength will come from. It comes from above.

Paul was fifty-one years old when I arrived at his door. He is now a remarkable eighty-three. I was a thirty-one-year-old woman and very ill. I am now a healthy, independent sixty-four-year-old woman. I have conquered many fears and obsessions. I feel more alive and vibrant at this age than I did at thirty.

As I finish this part of my memoir, it is 2011. I now create a bi-weekly cartoon, "My Duma," for a local newspaper, The Columbia Insider." I am an amateur photographer, who thoroughly enjoys shooting anything fascinating and, I might add, in all kinds of weather. I started a small company called Vona Ventures. The purpose of the business is to promote creativity through photography, writing and drawing. I sell a large assortment of greeting cards created from my photography. I also give computer lessons — Apple and PC. Temperature changes still affect me and the migraines continue. I do the best I can. I don't stop living; I shall overcome.

There was a time in my life when I felt as if the day dragged on forever, and the agony was close to unbearable at times. Now, I can't fit enough into each beautiful day. Every morning as I open my eyes, I am amazed at the glory of God's earth and all that's in front of me. I have a thirst to learn and grow and become totally whole and fulfilled from experiences and knowledge. As I seek out the treasures hidden in every day life I am inspired to give all of myself and hopefully enhance the space I take up.

God has blessed me beyond words. I was given a second chance. Occasionally, when I think back to when the addiction started, it is difficult to comprehend how far I have come. I can truly say I have my life back. It was always there. God just gave me the time and the tools to enjoy it once again.

Appendix

Hypothermia in a Patient
with Anorexia Nervosa
Diane K. Smith, Lars Ovesen, Richard Chu,
Stephen Sackel, and Lyn Howard

A young woman with anorexia nervosa had severe recurrent *hypothermia*. Initial evaluation revealed a *thiamine* deficiency. Administration of pharmacologic doses of thiamine improved voluntary food intake, and her temperature normalized. Following the restoration of body weight, withdrawal of supplemental thiamine produced a clinical relapse. After reinstitution of supplemental thiamine, the patient again became *asymptomatic* until she chose to consume a calorically restricted diet. With progressive weight loss, hypothermia recurred and was unresponsive to thiamine therapy. Fortuitously, the patient's intake of sucrose was abruptly increased, and her body temperature normalized within seven days. The potential roles of thiamine and carbohydrate in *thermoregulation* are discussed.

The patient was a 33-year old woman with a 10-year history of *anorexia nervosa* characterized by phases of mild obesity alternating with periods of severe self-induced starvation. One year before admission, mild hypothermia (rectal temperature 94.8 degrees F) was documented. At that time she weighed 62 % of her ideal body weight (IBW). In the subsequent months, she gained 75 lbs. (110% IBW) and initiated a 5-week fast. Thereafter, she ate about 1200 kcal/d, estimated to contain 0.5-1.0 mg of thiamine per day. Her weight loss during this interval was 35 lbs. Secondary *amenorrhea* recurred, and she became increasingly anorectic, weak, and heat intolerant. She denied intake of alcohol or drugs.

On admission, her rectal temperature was 88.0 degrees F., blood pressure 90/55, pulse 56 and regular, height 69 in, and weight 128 (87% IBW). Neurologic examination revealed constricted but reactive pupils, a fine resting tremor, and absent Achilles tendon reflexes. She appeared irritable and depressed but was alert and oriented with intact memory. Despite her low core temperature, her extremities felt warm to touch. She failed to exhibit rebound *tachycardia* following a *Valsalva's maneuver*, however, her heart rate increased in response to exercise. The remainder of the physical examination was unremarkable. The patient's hypothermia was attributed to cold exposure, since the external environmental temperature was 0-10 degrees F, and she reported taking ice baths to stimulate her appetite. For four days she received intravenous fluids containing 5 % dextrose, saline, and multivitamins that provided a total of 500 mg of thiamine hydrochloride. *Nasogastric* tube feedings was initiated on the fourth hospital day. Her body temperature normalized after five days, and she remained *euthermic* for eight additional days. Subsequently, her core temperature progressively fell to 92 degrees F, despite a room temperature of 68 degrees F, warming blankets, and 2000 kcal/d of nasogastric tube feedings. Hypothermia was verified by simultaneous temperature determinations of freshly voided urine. Consequently, a fixed hypothalamic lesion was considered. *Endocrine* evaluation showed intact thyroid and adrenal cortical function. One hour of cold exposure (59 degrees F) induced neither *vasoconstriction* nor shivering, whereas external warming (80 degrees F) resulted in peripheral *vasodilation* and a further fall in core temperature.

Treatment with 300 mg thiamine per day by mouth was initiated, and the body temperature normalized within six days. *Concomitantly*, there was a marked improvement in mood, heat tolerance, and appetite. Tube feeding was discontinued and satisfactory weight gain resulted. The patient was discharged on 300 mg thiamine per day.

Three months after discharge, after achieving her ideal body weight, the effect of thiamine withdrawal was assessed. Within 2 weeks, the patient complained of increasing anorexia and heat intolerance. The whole-blood thiamine level fell to 12 ng/ml, and transketolase stimulation rose to 100 %. Transketolase activity (reflecting apoenzyme concentration) was within the normal range. Thiamine supplementation was resumed and was associated with a prompt rise in blood thiamine levels and eventual normalization of transketolase stimulation after 8 months of thiamine supplementation. The patient ate heartily and again became mildly obese (169 lb.) To avoid a self-imposed fast, she was advised to follow a 1200-kcal balanced deficit diet. Despite continued supplementation with 300 mg thiamine per day, a fall in body temperature accompanied the ensuing weight loss and was recorded at 90 degrees F on several occasions by both the patient and trained personnel. Attempts to increase spontaneous caloric intake were resisted. The dosage of thiamine was empirically doubled, although blood thiamine values were persistently normal or elevated. After several episodes of severe disorientation accompanying *hypothermia,* her boyfriend removed all foods containing artificial sweeteners and replaced them with foods high in sucrose content. From dietary recalls it was estimated that her sucrose intake increased from 25 to 200 g/d. Rectal temperature normalized within seven days. Progressive weight gain ensued, again resulting in obesity (180 lb). In the past few months, the patient was observed in the hospital to experience uncontrollable carbohydrate binges (up to 7000 kcal/d) and mild *hyperthermia* (up to 100.0 degrees F) Withdrawal of thiamine supplementation has not altered her temperature or thiamine status. Attempts to modify her high caloric intake under hospital observation were resisted. We await her next self-imposed severe diet restriction to confirm our *hypothesis* that her hypothermia represents a fixed lesion, which is unresponsive to thiamine but controlled by dietary carbohydrate.

Reprinted with Permission
Licensee: Jill P Vona
License Date: Jul 26, 2011
License Number: 2716550492134
Licensed content publisher Elsevier
Elsevier VAT number GB 494 6272 12
The full case report can be obtained at http://www.sciencedirect.com/
Browse by title (M)
Metabolism (content-type journal)
Vol. 32 Art. 12
Hypothermia in a patient with anorexia nervosa
Pages 1151-1154
Diane K. Smith, Lars Ovesen, Richard Chu, Stephen Sackel, Lyn Howard
Albany Medical College, the Veterans Administration Medical
Center, Albany New York, USA 12208
Published by Elsevier Science, 1983
Corresponding Author: Dr. Lyn Howard
Supported by General Clinical Research Center grant number 1-MO-1-RR-0749-04 and USDA grant number 5901-0410-9-0297-0.

GLOSSARY

This glossary is to give the reader a better understanding of my interpretation of certain words. The following web sites are available for more specific information.

> 1-Dictionary: http://dictionary.reference.com
> 2-Wikipedia: http://en.wikipedia.org/wiki/Main_Page
> 3-Wiktionary: http://en.wiktionary.org/wiki/Wiktionary:Main_Page
> 4-Free Dictionary:
> http://medical-dictionary.thefreedictionary.com

Addiction - When something takes over a person's life where he or she feels a compulsive need to continue it daily in order to function and survive. (Emphasizing daily.) He or she *may* have a choice when the instance first begins or a need of physical relief. The person will do anything in their power to continue this obsessive *thing*. The addiction totally interferes with his or her life. They have no life. Their life becomes the compulsion. I believe that addictions go further than the medical definition. I question why the substance has to be a drug. Why can't it be the inhaling of cold air, or submersion into cold water, or ingesting cold liquids and cold food in a very cold environment? They will definitely cause an alteration in the brain. I engulfed my body in excessive cold temperatures for months. The result was a body temperature of 88°. When ice was taken away from me, I stopped eating for forty days. And without this cold I believed I was nothing. I barely functioned. I withdrew from society. I could not work, eat, or sleep without being in cold water. That was the most important thing in my life for sixteen years. If someone questions whether I was addicted or not, in my mind I will always believe that I was addicted to cold water.

Amenorrhoea-2 - Secondary amenorrhoea happens when a female stops having her period (menstrual cycle) for one reason or another. Sometimes it appears to be early menopause, but it can be other issues as well, such as sections in the brain may not be performing properly.

Anorexia nervosa-2 - Anorexia nervosa occurs when a person stops eating. When it goes on for a long period of time, usually the person involved is afraid of gaining too much weight and sees him or herself as overweight, even when they are not. Some people exercise to extreme and even take laxatives to get rid of any food intake. Without professional help, or a change in lifestyle, a victim of this disease can die.

Asymptomatic-1 - Shows no signs of being ill.

Concomitantly-3 - Two things are happening at the same time.

Endocrine-2 - The endocrine system plays a very important role in the body's metabolism. It can affect a person's mood swings plus many parts of the body. A patient feels like their entire body is out of balance. They just don't feel good. They are extremely tired and it is an effort to move. The skin can be dry and the hair brittle. Usually the patient knows that the body just isn't working properly.

Apoenzyme-2 - This is another word for enzymes.

Euthermic-4 - This is the process of becoming warm.

Hypothermia-2 - Hypothermia is when the body loses heat. The body core needs to be warm. Most of our heat loss is through the top of our head. When the body is cold, the blood vessels constrict. And the blood moves away from the extremities. It is traveling to the brain in order to preserve it. The brain is protected first. When the body continues to lose heat and the organs are unable to replenish this heat, then there isn't enough insulation on the brain and hypothermia sets in. The body temperature plummets; the patient becomes incoherent or confused. The term I use is *spacey*.

Hyperthermia-2 - Hyperthermia is when the body becomes too warm and it cannot get rid of the heat, which can then lead to heat stroke.

Hypothalamic-2 - In order to describe hypothalamic it is necessary to understand the function of the **hypothalamus**. It controls a person's desire for food and liquids, which in turn controls the body temperature. How a person sleeps and their emotional state is part of the hypothalamus.

Hypothesis-2 - A scientific hypothesis predicts what will come of a test or experiment not performed yet. The outcome isn't certified as yet. There is more work to be done before it becomes a true observation that can be documented and then followed by others.

Nasogastric intubation-2 - This is the process of putting a plastic tube into the body so that food can be passed through the tube to feed a patient. One way is to put the tube through the nose, and then it must pass through the throat and eventually land in the stomach. Often an x-ray is taken to make sure it doesn't get placed in the lung by mistake

Obsession - When a person is preoccupied with a repetitive behavior that interferes with his or her life, and what most people consider abnormal. An idea or feeling that preoccupies the mind to the extent of being destructive.

Raynaud's Syndrome - This is a condition where the fingers turn white. It usually happens because they are exposed to cold. The body wants to protect its inner core and very important organs from severe damage, so it draws the blood from the extremities. The blood leaves the fingers and in turn, they lose the normal color. It is also quite painful. When the blood is rushing back into the fingers, they turn a bluish color. This is somewhat uncomfortable as well, until the hands are back to their normal state. Someone with this syndrome can have their fingers turn white just by putting their hands in the refrigerator freezer section. Stress can also bring it on along with temperature changes.

Ritual - When a person creates a repetitive pattern, which they feel, enhances their day.

Tachycardia-3 - A person can be sitting still with no exertion and their heart rate is beating much too fast.

Thermoregulation-2 - If a person's surroundings are much different from his or her own body temperature and the body can maintain a normal body temperature that is thermoregulation. When the body overheats it has a heat stroke, and when it becomes too cold the body is in a state of hypothermia.

<u>**Thiamin**</u> or **thiamine**-2 - A vitamin. If a person is low in thiamine it can lead to weight loss, confusion and bad mood swings. Severe cases can affect the heart and nervous system.

<u>**Transketolase-2**</u> - An enzyme. If this enzyme is reduced, then the thiamin level is affected and the outcome can lead to malnutrition.

<u>**Valsalva maneuver-2**</u> - Look up on the Internet or ask a physician.

<u>**Vasoconstriction-2**</u> - When the blood vessels become smaller or slender.

<u>**Vasodilation-2**</u> - The opposite of vasoconstriction. When the blood vessels become larger or expand.

BIBLIOGRAPHY

Amplified Bible, Expanded Edition. Zondervan Corporation and Lockman Foundation, 1987.

Anonymous. "Rainbow Bridge."

Chicago. Rock-and-roll band. Chicago, 1967.

Cox-Chapman, Mally. The Case for Heaven: Near Death Experiences as Evidence of the Afterlife. New York: G.P. Putnam's Sons, 1995.

"Duma." Pro. Gaylord Films, 2005. DVD

Easton, Sheena. "Morning Train." 1981.

Hospital Photos of Jill Peck. Courtesy of Albany Medical Center, Albany, New York.

Lawrence, D. H. Lady Chatterley's Lover. Florence, Italy: private publication, 1928.

Lili. MGM, 1953. VHS.

M*A*S*H. Twentieth Century Fox for CBS, 1972, TV Series.

McWhirter, Norris, and Ross McWhirter. The Guinness Book of Records. London, 1955.

"Quotes of His Holiness the Dalai Lama of Tibet." Brainy Quotes http://www.brainyquote.com/quotes/authors/d/dalai_lama.html.

Simmons, Richard. Reach. Elektra, 1982.

Smith, Diane K. et al., Metabolism. "Hypothermia in a Patient with Anorexia Nervosa." December 1983. pp.1151-1154.

Southey, Robert. Goldilocks and the Three Bears. England, 1837.

Things We Lost in the Fire. DreamWorks, 2007. DVD.

Travers, P. L. Mary Poppins. England, 1934.

Weiss, Donna, and Jackie DeShannon. "Betty Davis Eyes." 1974.

ABOUT THE AUTHOR

Born in Massachusetts and raised in Copake, New York, Jill Peck Vona now resides in Latham, New York.

In 2009, she formed a small company. Vona Ventures, a greeting card line, displays Jill's photography.

In 2011, Jill received the Reader's Digest Bronze Award for an earlier edition of her story.

Jill's cartoon series, "My Duma", is published bi-weekly in a local newspaper.

Jill can be reached by e-mail at peckvona@gmail.com. Check out her website located at www.jillpeckvonaphotography.com or https://sites.google.com/site/vonaventures64/

CPSIA information can be obtained at www.ICGtesting.com
Printed in the USA
BVOW012258190213

313725BV00021B/657/P